The Natural Path to Healing Your Nervous System

Luna Parnell

Table of Content

Legal Disclaimer

The information provided in **The Natural Path to Healing Your Nervous System** is for educational and informational purposes only and is not intended as medical advice. This book is not a substitute for professional medical diagnosis, treatment, or care. Always consult with a qualified healthcare provider before beginning any new treatment regimen, including herbal, vitamin, mineral, or dietary supplements.

The author and publisher are not responsible for any adverse effects or consequences resulting from the use of any suggestions or information contained within this book. Individual results may vary, and the use of natural remedies should be tailored to your specific health needs, considering any existing medical conditions or medications. Never disregard professional medical advice or delay seeking it because of something you have read in this book.

By reading this book, you acknowledge that the author and publisher are not liable for any health decisions you make based on the content herein. Always seek professional advice before making changes to your health care practices.

Introduction

The nervous system is the intricate, awe-inspiring control center of our body—a network of communication that connects every sensation, thought, and movement. It is a system that never rests, constantly processing and responding to both the outside world and the inner workings of our bodies. From the simple reflexes that keep us safe to the complex functions that govern our emotions, cognition, and voluntary actions, the nervous system is at the heart of everything we do.

In today's fast-paced world, our nervous systems are often under more strain than ever before. Stress, poor diet, lack of sleep, environmental toxins, and even emotional turmoil can all take their toll, disrupting the delicate balance necessary for optimal health. When this system is compromised, the effects ripple through the entire body, leading to issues like anxiety, depression, chronic pain, fatigue, and impaired cognitive function. Yet, just as the nervous system has a remarkable capacity for adaptation, it also holds a great potential for healing.

This book, *The Natural Path to Healing Your Nervous System*, is a guide to understanding and nurturing the very foundation of your body's communication network. We will explore the intricate anatomy of the nervous system, from the brain and spinal cord to the far-reaching nerves that regulate every organ and muscle. But more importantly, we'll dive into natural ways to support, protect, and restore its health.

Through the integration of herbal remedies, vitamins, minerals, and supplements, alongside lifestyle adjustments, you'll learn how to balance and rejuvenate your nervous system. Whether you're seeking to reduce stress, enhance brain function, or simply promote overall well-being, this journey will provide the tools you need to support your body's most vital system.

In embarking on this path, we return to nature's wisdom—choosing gentle, effective methods that align with the body's inherent capacity to heal. This is a journey not just of science, but of holistic understanding, bringing together ancient knowledge and modern research. Your nervous system is the key to your body's vitality, and the path to healing begins here.

Nervous System Overview:

The nervous system is divided into two main parts:

1. **Central Nervous System (CNS):** This includes the brain and spinal cord, which act as the control center for processing and sending out information.
2. **Peripheral Nervous System (PNS):** This comprises the nerves that extend from the brain and spinal cord to the rest of the body, including the limbs and organs. It is further divided into the somatic and autonomic nervous systems.

Components of the Nervous System:

1. **Neurons (Nerve Cells):**
   - The fundamental units of the nervous system that transmit electrical signals. Each neuron has three parts:
     - **Cell body (Soma):** Contains the nucleus and is the neuron's metabolic center.
     - **Dendrites:** Branch-like structures that receive

signals from other neurons.

- **Axon:** A long projection that transmits signals to other neurons, muscles, or glands.

2. **Brain:**
   - The central organ of the CNS is responsible for processing information and controlling functions like thought, emotion, movement, and sensory perception. The brain is divided into various regions:
     - **Cerebrum:** Controls voluntary activities, speech, thought, memory, and emotion.
     - **Cerebellum:** Coordinates movement, balance, and posture.
     - **Brainstem:** Regulates vital functions like breathing, heart rate, and digestion.

3. **Spinal Cord:**
   - A long, thin bundle of nerves that runs from the brain down through the spine. It transmits

signals between the brain and the body and plays a role in reflex actions.

4. **Peripheral Nerves:**
    - These nerves branch out from the CNS to the rest of the body. They carry sensory information to the CNS and transmit motor commands from the CNS to muscles and glands.

Divisions of the Peripheral Nervous System:

- **Somatic Nervous System:** Controls voluntary movements by connecting the CNS to skeletal muscles.
- **Autonomic Nervous System (ANS):** Controls involuntary functions, such as heart rate, digestion, and respiratory rate. It is divided into:
    - **Sympathetic Nervous System:** Prepares the body for "fight or flight" during stressful situations.
    - **Parasympathetic Nervous System:** Promotes "rest and

digest" activities, conserving energy and promoting relaxation.

Nerve Impulses and Synapses:

- **Nerve Impulse:** Electrical signals that travel along neurons, allowing for communication between different parts of the body.
- **Synapse:** The junction between two neurons where neurotransmitters are released to relay signals.

Neurotransmitters:

- **Dopamine, Serotonin, Acetylcholine, and GABA** are examples of chemical messengers that neurons use to communicate across synapses. Each neurotransmitter has a different role in regulating mood, movement, cognition, and other functions.

Reflexes:

- **Reflex Arc:** A simple nerve pathway involved in reflex actions, which are rapid, involuntary responses to stimuli, like pulling your hand away from a hot surface.

Nervous System Function:

- **Sensory Input:** Detects changes in the environment (internal and external) through sensory organs and receptors.
- **Integration:** The CNS processes the sensory information and determines the appropriate response.
- **Motor Output:** Sends signals to muscles or glands to carry out the response.

The nervous system is integral to how our body perceives the world and reacts to it. It manages both conscious actions and unconscious physiological processes, ensuring we can interact with our environment and maintain internal balance.

Central Nervous System (CNS)

The **Central Nervous System (CNS)** is the core of the body's nervous system, consisting of two primary components: the **brain** and the **spinal cord**. Together, these structures are responsible for processing and transmitting information throughout the body. The CNS acts as the control center, interpreting sensory data from the external environment and coordinating responses that regulate body functions, including movement, thought, and emotional responses.

Brain

The brain is the command center of the CNS, composed of billions of neurons that communicate through intricate networks. It controls cognitive functions, motor skills, sensory perception, and emotions. The brain is divided into several key regions:

- **Cerebrum**: The largest part, responsible for conscious thought, memory, and voluntary muscle movement.

- **Cerebellum**: Involved in balance, posture, and coordination of movements.
- **Brainstem**: Regulates essential life functions such as breathing, heart rate, and sleep cycles.

Spinal Cord

The spinal cord is a long, cylindrical structure that extends from the brainstem down through the vertebral column. It acts as a communication highway, transmitting signals between the brain and the rest of the body. It also controls reflexes and automatic responses to stimuli that do not require brain involvement.

Functions of the CNS

The primary role of the CNS is to integrate information from the peripheral nervous system and make decisions about how the body should respond. Key functions include:

- **Sensory Processing**: Interpreting input from the senses (touch, sight, sound, taste, and smell).
- **Motor Control**: Initiating and controlling muscle movements.

- **Cognitive Functions**: Memory, reasoning, problem-solving, and learning.
- **Regulation of Internal Systems**: Controlling vital functions such as blood pressure, heart rate, and body temperature.

The CNS is protected by layers of membranes called the **meninges** and by the **cerebrospinal fluid (CSF)**, which cushions the brain and spinal cord. However, it is also vulnerable to injuries, diseases, and degenerative conditions.

Herbs

1. **Ginkgo Biloba**: Increases blood flow to the brain, improves memory, and may protect against neurodegenerative diseases.
2. **Ashwagandha**: Known for reducing stress and supporting brain health by protecting nerve cells from oxidative damage.
3. **Bacopa Monnieri**: Traditionally used for cognitive enhancement, memory improvement, and supporting neuroplasticity.

4. **Gotu Kola**: Supports circulation to the brain, promotes cognitive function, and may help with anxiety.

Vitamins

1. **Vitamin B12**: Essential for nerve health and the production of myelin, the protective sheath around nerves.
2. **Vitamin D**: Supports brain health and mood regulation, and protects against neurodegenerative diseases.
3. **Vitamin E**: Acts as an antioxidant, protecting brain cells from oxidative stress and supporting long-term cognitive function.
4. **Vitamin B6**: Plays a key role in neurotransmitter function and helps maintain healthy nerve signaling.

Minerals

1. **Magnesium**: Essential for nerve function, it helps regulate neurotransmitters and can protect against brain inflammation.
2. **Zinc**: Plays a role in cognitive function, and memory formation, and is involved in nerve signaling.

3. **Iron**: Important for oxygen transport to the brain and for the production of neurotransmitters.
4. **Selenium**: Acts as an antioxidant that helps protect the nervous system from damage caused by oxidative stress.

Supplements

1. **Omega-3 Fatty Acids (EPA/DHA)**: Crucial for brain function, these fats support cognitive health and protect against brain aging.
2. **Acetyl-L-Carnitine**: Supports energy production in brain cells and can improve memory and focus.
3. **Phosphatidylserine**: Aids in protecting brain cells and improving cognitive performance, especially memory.
4. **Alpha-Lipoic Acid**: An antioxidant that helps reduce oxidative stress and supports overall nerve health.

These natural treatments, combined with proper diet and lifestyle choices, can promote the regeneration, maintenance, and overall health of the central nervous system, helping to preserve cognitive function and protect against neurological decline.

Peripheral Nervous System (PNS)

The **Peripheral Nervous System (PNS)** is a crucial part of the overall nervous system, consisting of all the nerves that lie outside the brain and spinal cord. Its primary function is to connect the central nervous system (CNS) — which includes the brain and spinal cord — to the rest of the body, such as limbs, organs, and skin. This allows the PNS to relay information between the CNS and the external environment, as well as internal bodily processes.

Key Functions of the PNS

1. **Sensory Function (Afferent Pathways)**: The PNS gathers sensory information from the external environment and internal organs, sending this data to the CNS for interpretation. Sensory nerves detect stimuli like temperature, pain, touch, and body position (proprioception).
2. **Motor Function (Efferent Pathways)**: Once the CNS processes

information, the PNS sends motor commands back to muscles and glands, coordinating voluntary movements (such as walking) and involuntary actions (such as heart rate and digestion).

Components of the PNS

1. **Cranial Nerves**: There are 12 pairs of cranial nerves that emerge directly from the brain and brainstem, handling sensory and motor functions in areas such as the head, neck, and upper body. For example, the optic nerve is responsible for vision, while the vagus nerve regulates heart and digestive functions.
2. **Spinal Nerves**: There are 31 pairs of spinal nerves that branch out from the spinal cord, serving different parts of the body. These nerves are responsible for both sensory input (feeling) and motor output (movement).
3. **Autonomic Nervous System (ANS)**: A division of the PNS, the autonomic system controls involuntary functions such as heart rate, digestion, and respiratory rate. It consists of:

- ○ **Sympathetic Nervous System**: Prepares the body for "fight or flight" responses during stress or danger, increasing heart rate and blood flow to muscles.
  - ○ **Parasympathetic Nervous System**: Promotes "rest and digest" activities, conserving energy, and returning the body to a state of calm after a stressful situation.
4. **Somatic Nervous System**: Another division of the PNS, the somatic system is responsible for voluntary movements, relaying signals from the CNS to skeletal muscles and coordinating conscious motor activity like walking, running, or grasping objects.

Structure of the PNS

- **Nerves**: The main component of the PNS, nerves are bundles of axons (nerve fibers) that carry electrical impulses. They can be either:
  - ○ **Sensory (Afferent) Nerves**: Transmit information from sensory receptors (like skin or eyes) to the CNS.

- o **Motor (Efferent) Nerves**: Carry instructions from the CNS to muscles and glands.
  - o **Mixed Nerves**: Contain both sensory and motor fibers, performing both functions simultaneously.
- **Ganglia**: Clusters of nerve cell bodies in the PNS that act as relay stations, processing sensory and motor signals.

The Role of the PNS in Reflexes

Reflexes are automatic, rapid responses to stimuli, such as pulling your hand away from a hot object. The PNS plays a key role in reflex arcs, bypassing the brain to provide a quick response via the spinal cord. This helps protect the body from harm by reacting faster than if the brain were involved.

Disorders of the PNS

Damage or dysfunction in the PNS can result in peripheral neuropathy, which can cause symptoms like numbness, tingling, weakness, and pain. Causes of PNS disorders include diabetes, infections, trauma, and toxins. Maintaining PNS health is essential for overall body function and response to stimuli.

The PNS plays an indispensable role in keeping the body connected to the CNS, ensuring we can perceive and react to the world around us while maintaining essential bodily functions.

Herbs

1. **St. John's Wort**: Traditionally used to alleviate nerve pain and improve mood, it can support peripheral nerve health.
2. **Skullcap**: Known for its ability to calm the nervous system, it helps with nerve regeneration and reduces neuropathic pain.
3. **Lion's Mane Mushroom**: Promotes nerve growth factor (NGF), supporting the regeneration and repair of peripheral nerves.
4. **Valerian Root**: Helps soothe the nerves and may reduce nerve-related pain, particularly in cases of sciatica.

Vitamins

1. **Vitamin B1 (Thiamine)**: Vital for nerve function and energy metabolism, it helps prevent nerve damage, especially in conditions like neuropathy.

2. **Vitamin B5 (Pantothenic Acid)**: Plays a key role in nerve signaling and the production of neurotransmitters.
3. **Vitamin B9 (Folate)**: Supports nerve cell function and repair by aiding in the synthesis of DNA and RNA.
4. **Vitamin B7 (Biotin)**: Important for nerve health and metabolic support, especially in maintaining the myelin sheath.

Minerals

1. **Calcium**: Essential for nerve transmission and muscle contractions, helping ensure proper communication between the nervous system and muscles.
2. **Copper**: Involved in maintaining healthy nerve tissues and supports the production of neurotransmitters.
3. **Potassium**: Important for the conduction of electrical signals in the peripheral nervous system, helping with nerve and muscle communication.
4. **Manganese**: Supports antioxidant defense systems in nerve cells and is involved in nerve signal transmission.

Supplements

1. **Coenzyme Q10**: Protects nerve cells from oxidative damage and helps with energy production, especially in peripheral nerves.
2. **N-Acetyl Cysteine (NAC)**: Promotes glutathione production, supporting antioxidant defenses in the nervous system and aiding in nerve repair.
3. **Lipoic Acid**: Helps to regenerate nerves, particularly in diabetic neuropathy, and reduces oxidative stress.
4. **Gamma-Linolenic Acid (GLA)**: Found in evening primrose oil, it helps with nerve regeneration and reduces inflammation in the peripheral nerves.

These nutrients support nerve regeneration, reduce oxidative stress, improve nerve communication, and promote overall peripheral nervous system health. This natural approach can aid in preventing and healing nerve damage, enhancing nerve function, and promoting long-term nerve vitality.

Neurons (Nerve Cells)

Neurons are the fundamental units of the nervous system, responsible for transmitting and processing information throughout the body. They are specialized cells designed to carry electrical and chemical signals, making them vital for communication within the nervous system. Each neuron consists of three primary components: the cell body (soma), dendrites, and an axon.

Structure of a Neuron:

1. **Cell Body (Soma)**: The cell body contains the nucleus, which houses the genetic material of the neuron. It also contains other organelles essential for the cell's metabolic activities, such as the production of neurotransmitters. The soma integrates signals received from the dendrites.
2. **Dendrites**: These are tree-like structures that branch out from the cell body. Dendrites receive signals from other neurons and transmit them to the soma. The more extensive the dendritic network, the more signals the neuron can receive.

3. **Axon**: The axon is a long, slender projection that transmits signals away from the cell body toward other neurons, muscles, or glands. Some axons can be as long as a meter. At the end of the axon are axon terminals, which release neurotransmitters that communicate with the next cell.
4. **Myelin Sheath**: Many axons are covered by a fatty layer called the myelin sheath. This insulating layer speeds up the transmission of electrical signals along the axon. Myelin is produced by glial cells (Schwann cells in the PNS and oligodendrocytes in the CNS).
5. **Synapse**: This is the junction between the axon terminal of one neuron and the dendrite or cell body of another neuron. Signals are passed across the synapse via chemical messengers known as neurotransmitters.

Types of Neurons:

1. **Sensory Neurons (Afferent)**: These neurons carry information from sensory receptors (e.g., skin, eyes, ears) toward the CNS for processing.
2. **Motor Neurons (Efferent)**: These neurons carry instructions from the CNS

to muscles and glands, controlling voluntary and involuntary actions.

3. **Interneurons**: These neurons act as connectors or relays within the CNS, linking sensory and motor neurons and helping to process information.

Function of Neurons:

- Neurons communicate through electrical impulses called action potentials. When a neuron receives a signal strong enough to reach a certain threshold, an action potential is generated. This electrical impulse travels down the axon to the axon terminal, where it triggers the release of neurotransmitters into the synapse. The neurotransmitters bind to receptors on the next cell, transmitting the signal.

Role of Neurons in Reflexes:

Neurons are integral to reflex arcs. Sensory neurons detect stimuli and send signals to the spinal cord, where interneurons process the information. The response is transmitted to motor neurons, which control muscle contractions, enabling rapid, automatic reactions like pulling your hand away from a flame.

Herbs, Vitamins, Minerals, and Supplements (HVMS) for Neuron Health:

1. **Herbs:**
   - **Ginkgo Biloba**: Known for its potential to enhance cognitive function and improve blood circulation in the brain, Ginkgo Biloba supports the health of neurons by increasing oxygen and nutrient supply.
   - **Bacopa Monnieri**: This herb is recognized for its neuroprotective properties and is often used to improve memory and cognitive function by reducing oxidative stress on neurons.
   - **Ashwagandha**: Traditionally used in Ayurveda, ashwagandha helps reduce stress and anxiety, which can support overall neuron function and mental clarity.
   - **Gotu Kola**: Another adaptogenic herb that promotes brain

function, improves circulation and may help repair nerve damage.

2. **Vitamins:**
    - **Vitamin B12**: Essential for maintaining the myelin sheath that insulates axons and supports nerve regeneration. Deficiency in B12 can lead to nerve damage and cognitive impairments.
    - **Vitamin B6**: Vital for neurotransmitter synthesis, including serotonin and dopamine, B6 aids neuron communication and mental well-being.
    - **Vitamin D**: Supports nerve growth and development, particularly in the central nervous system. It also plays a role in reducing inflammation, which can protect neurons from damage.

3. **Minerals:**
    - **Magnesium**: Important for nerve signal transmission and reducing neuronal excitability. It helps in the relaxation of nerves

and muscles and is beneficial in maintaining brain health.

- **Zinc**: Critical for synaptic plasticity, zinc supports proper neurotransmitter function and is involved in regulating communication between neurons.
- **Calcium**: Plays a crucial role in neurotransmitter release and muscle contraction. Adequate calcium levels are needed for neuron communication and overall nervous system function.

4. **Supplements:**

- **Omega-3 Fatty Acids (DHA & EPA)**: Omega-3s are key components of neuron membranes and are essential for proper brain function and development. DHA supports neuron structure, while EPA helps reduce inflammation.
- **Acetyl-L-Carnitine**: This supplement promotes mitochondrial health and energy production in neurons, helping to protect against neurodegeneration and improve cognitive function.

- **Alpha-Lipoic Acid**: An antioxidant that helps protect neurons from oxidative damage and may enhance nerve function and regeneration.

Maintaining neuron health is vital for the proper functioning of the entire nervous system, and supporting them with the right herbs, vitamins, minerals, and supplements can improve cognitive function, reduce stress, and protect against neurodegenerative conditions.

Cell Body (Soma)

The **cell body**, also known as the **soma**, is the central part of a neuron. It contains the nucleus and other vital organelles, making it responsible for the metabolic functions of the neuron. The soma is crucial for the cell's health, maintenance, and function, as it integrates incoming signals from the dendrites and generates the necessary biochemical components for neural communication.

Components of the Soma:

1. **Nucleus**: The nucleus houses the neuron's genetic material (DNA). It is the control center of the cell, regulating gene expression and overseeing cell activity, including protein synthesis. The proteins made in the soma are essential for neuron structure and function.
2. **Cytoplasm**: The fluid that fills the soma, containing various organelles such as mitochondria, ribosomes, and the Golgi apparatus. The cytoplasm facilitates biochemical reactions that support the neuron's activity.
3. **Mitochondria**: These are the energy producers of the cell, generating ATP

(adenosine triphosphate) through cellular respiration. Since neurons have high energy demands due to constant signaling, mitochondria are essential for maintaining their functionality.

4. **Endoplasmic Reticulum (ER)**: The rough ER is responsible for protein synthesis, while the smooth ER plays a role in lipid synthesis and calcium storage. The proteins produced in the rough ER are crucial for maintaining the structure of the neuron and its communication capabilities.

5. **Golgi Apparatus**: This organelle modifies, sorts, and packages proteins and lipids for transport to other parts of the neuron, including the axon and dendrites. It plays a key role in preparing neurotransmitters for synaptic transmission.

6. **Nissl Bodies**: These are clusters of rough endoplasmic reticulum and ribosomes within the soma, specifically involved in the production of proteins necessary for the growth and repair of neurons.

7. **Cytoskeleton**: The soma contains a network of microtubules and filaments that provide structural support to the

cell and aid in the transport of materials throughout the neuron. The cytoskeleton is crucial for maintaining the shape of the neuron and for axonal transport, which is the movement of proteins and organelles down the axon to the synapse.

Functions of the Soma:

- **Integration of Signals**: The soma processes electrical impulses received from the dendrites. If the cumulative signals reach a threshold, the soma initiates an action potential that travels down the axon to communicate with other neurons or muscles.
- **Metabolic Activity**: The soma is responsible for all the metabolic processes necessary for neuron survival, including energy production, protein synthesis, and waste removal. It ensures that the neuron has the resources to transmit signals efficiently.
- **Maintenance and Repair**: Neurons have limited regenerative capabilities, but the soma plays a vital role in maintaining the neuron's health by producing the proteins and enzymes required for repair.

Herbs, Vitamins, Minerals, and Supplements (HVMS) for Soma Health:

1. **Herbs**:
   - **Rhodiola Rosea**: Known for its adaptogenic properties, Rhodiola helps improve energy production in cells and reduces oxidative stress, protecting neurons.
   - **Lion's Mane Mushroom**: Supports neurogenesis and has been shown to promote the growth of new nerve cells, aiding in the repair and maintenance of neurons.
   - **Turmeric (Curcumin)**: A potent anti-inflammatory and antioxidant that protects the soma from oxidative stress and may reduce neuroinflammation.
2. **Vitamins**:
   - **Vitamin B12**: Crucial for neuron health and the production of myelin, vitamin B12 supports DNA synthesis and repair, as well as overall neuron maintenance.
   - **Vitamin E**: An antioxidant that protects neurons from oxidative damage by neutralizing free

radicals, supporting the longevity
and functionality of the soma.

   o **Vitamin C**: Important for
      collagen production, vitamin C
      supports the structural integrity
      of neurons and protects them
      from oxidative stress.

3. **Minerals**:

   o **Magnesium**: Essential for
      numerous biochemical reactions
      in the body, magnesium supports
      neuronal function by aiding in
      energy production and regulating
      neurotransmitter release.

   o **Selenium**: Acts as an
      antioxidant and is important for
      neuron protection, as it helps
      prevent oxidative damage that
      can affect the cell body.

   o **Copper**: Required for the
      formation of neurotransmitters
      and proper brain function, copper
      plays a role in maintaining the
      overall health of the neuron.

4. **Supplements**:

   o **Coenzyme Q10 (CoQ10)**: This
      antioxidant is involved in energy
      production within the
      mitochondria, helping the soma

meet its high energy demands and protecting it from oxidative damage.

- **Phosphatidylserine**: A phospholipid that helps maintain cell membrane integrity, particularly in neurons, and supports cognitive function by enhancing neuron communication.
- **N-Acetyl Cysteine (NAC)**: An antioxidant that boosts glutathione levels, NAC helps protect neurons from oxidative stress and supports cellular health.

The health and function of the soma are integral to the overall activity of neurons and the nervous system. Supporting the soma with proper nutrients can ensure effective neuronal communication and long-term cognitive health.

Dendrites

Dendrites are the branched extensions of a neuron that receive signals from other neurons and relay them to the cell body (soma). They play a critical role in neural communication, as they are the primary structures that bring information into the neuron, processing the signals received from other cells in the nervous system. Dendrites are highly specialized for receiving synaptic inputs and can have thousands of branches, each forming connections with other neurons.

Structure and Components:

1. **Dendritic Tree**: The complex, tree-like structure of dendrites increases the surface area of the neuron, allowing it to form more synapses with other neurons. This branching maximizes the amount of information a neuron can receive.
2. **Dendritic Spines**: Tiny protrusions along the dendrites where synapses form. Each spine serves as a site of synaptic transmission, connecting to an axon terminal from another neuron. Dendritic spines are dynamic structures that can change in shape and density,

which is important for learning and memory.

3. **Receptors**: Embedded within the membrane of dendrites are various receptor proteins that respond to neurotransmitters released by neighboring neurons. These receptors trigger electrical or chemical signals inside the neuron once they are activated by specific neurotransmitters.

4. **Microtubules and Actin Filaments**: Inside dendrites, the cytoskeleton is composed of microtubules and actin filaments. Microtubules assist in the transport of molecular cargo, such as proteins and organelles, while actin filaments are crucial for maintaining dendritic spine structure and plasticity.

5. **Ion Channels**: Dendrites are equipped with various ion channels, which allow the flow of ions such as sodium, potassium, and calcium. These ion channels regulate the electrical activity within the dendrite, playing a key role in how signals are transmitted to the soma.

Function of Dendrites:

- **Signal Reception**: Dendrites receive chemical signals (neurotransmitters) from the axon terminals of other neurons at synapses. These signals are converted into electrical impulses, known as postsynaptic potentials, which travel towards the soma.

- **Signal Integration**: Dendrites integrate the incoming signals from multiple sources. If the cumulative electrical activity is strong enough, it triggers an action potential in the soma, which is then transmitted down the axon.
- **Synaptic Plasticity**: Dendrites and their spines exhibit plasticity, meaning they can strengthen or weaken synaptic connections in response to experience or learning. This plasticity is key for memory formation and neural adaptation.
- **Processing Information**: Beyond simple transmission, dendrites also play an active role in processing information, as certain types of dendrites can initiate local action potentials (dendritic spikes), influencing how neurons respond to stimuli.

Herbs, Vitamins, Minerals, and Supplements (HVMS) for Dendrite Health:

1. **Herbs**:
   - **Ginkgo Biloba**: Known for improving blood flow to the brain, Ginkgo Biloba enhances cognitive function and supports neural plasticity, promoting healthy dendritic growth.
   - **Bacopa Monnieri**: An adaptogenic herb that supports memory and learning, Bacopa has been shown to promote dendritic branching and synapse formation.
   - **Ashwagandha**: Reduces oxidative stress and has neuroprotective properties, supporting dendritic growth and synaptic connections.
2. **Vitamins**:
   - **Vitamin D**: Essential for overall brain function, vitamin D supports synaptic plasticity and helps in the maintenance of dendritic structure.

- **Vitamin B6**: Important for neurotransmitter synthesis, vitamin B6 plays a role in neural communication and supports dendrite function by enhancing synaptic efficiency.
- **Folate (Vitamin B9)**: Crucial for DNA synthesis and repair, folate supports dendritic growth, neural development, and plasticity.

3. **Minerals**:

- **Zinc**: Plays a role in synaptic plasticity and neural communication. Zinc helps regulate the activity of neurotransmitter receptors, supporting dendrite function.
- **Calcium**: Vital for synaptic signaling, calcium ions trigger the release of neurotransmitters at synapses and help regulate the strength of synaptic connections in dendrites.
- **Magnesium**: Acts as a natural calcium channel blocker, helping to regulate synaptic activity and protect dendrites from excitotoxicity (overstimulation).

4. **Supplements**:
   - ○ **Omega-3 Fatty Acids (DHA)**: DHA is a critical component of neuronal membranes and supports dendrite growth, synapse formation, and plasticity, enhancing cognitive function.
   - ○ **N-Acetyl Cysteine (NAC)**: NAC boosts levels of glutathione, an antioxidant that protects neurons and dendrites from oxidative damage and supports dendritic function.
   - ○ **Phosphatidylserine**: A phospholipid that supports cell membrane integrity and enhances synaptic function, contributing to healthier dendritic networks.

Supporting dendrites with proper nutrients and herbs helps ensure that neural communication remains efficient and that the brain can adapt and respond to new information effectively. Healthy dendrites are essential for learning, memory, and overall cognitive function.

Axon

The **axon** is a long, slender projection of a neuron that transmits electrical impulses away from the neuron's cell body (soma) towards other neurons, muscles, or glands. Axons are fundamental to neural communication, as they are responsible for carrying action potentials (nerve impulses) from the neuron to its target cells. These impulses allow the brain and nervous system to control bodily functions and coordinate responses to stimuli.

Structure and Components:

1. **Axon Hillock**: The part of the soma where the axon originates. It is a critical area where the neuron integrates incoming signals and determines whether to initiate an action potential. If the cumulative input from the dendrites reaches a certain threshold, the axon hillock generates an action potential.
2. **Myelin Sheath**: In many neurons, the axon is wrapped in a fatty insulating layer called the myelin sheath, which is formed by **Schwann cells** in the peripheral nervous system or **oligodendrocytes** in the central nervous system. Myelin enhances the

speed of electrical signal transmission by allowing the action potential to jump between gaps in the myelin, known as the **Nodes of Ranvier**.

3. **Nodes of Ranvier**: These are small, unmyelinated sections of the axon where ion channels are concentrated. The action potential "jumps" from one node to the next in a process called **saltatory conduction**, which increases the speed of signal transmission.

4. **Axon Terminals (Synaptic Boutons)**: The axon ends in a series of branches that form synapses with target cells. Each branch ends in a terminal button or synaptic bouton, which contains neurotransmitters that are released in response to an action potential, allowing the neuron to communicate with other cells.

5. **Axoplasm**: The cytoplasm within the axon. It contains essential cellular components like mitochondria, microtubules, and other proteins required for the transport of substances along the axon, as well as for maintaining its structure and function.

6. **Axonal Transport**: Axons have a specialized system for transporting

materials between the soma and the axon terminals. This system includes **anterograde transport** (moving materials from the soma to the terminals) and **retrograde transport** (moving materials back to the soma).

The function of the Axon:

- **Action Potential Transmission**: The axon's primary role is to conduct action potentials from the soma to the synaptic terminals. Once the axon hillock generates an action potential, the electrical signal travels down the axon toward the axon terminals, where it will trigger the release of neurotransmitters.
- **Neurotransmitter Release**: When the action potential reaches the axon terminals, it causes calcium ions to enter the synaptic boutons, prompting the release of neurotransmitters into the synapse. These chemical signals cross the synapse and bind to receptors on the target cell, continuing the communication process.
- **Signal Amplification and Transmission Speed**: Axons ensure that signals can be transmitted rapidly and efficiently across long distances

within the nervous system. Myelinated axons, in particular, allow for the rapid conduction of electrical impulses, making communication between the brain and peripheral organs almost instantaneous.

Types of Axons:

- **Myelinated Axons**: These axons have a myelin sheath, which increases the speed of signal transmission. Myelinated axons are commonly found in neurons that need to transmit signals quickly, such as those controlling motor functions.
- **Unmyelinated Axons**: These axons lack a myelin sheath and conduct impulses more slowly. They are often found in parts of the nervous system where speed is less critical, such as certain sensory neurons.

Importance of Axons:

Axons are essential for connecting different parts of the nervous system and facilitating communication between neurons and their target cells, whether they are other neurons, muscle cells, or glands. Any damage to axons can disrupt neural communication, leading to neurological disorders or impaired motor function.

Herbs, Vitamins, Minerals, and Supplements (HVMS) for Axon Health:

1. **Herbs**:
   - **Lion's Mane Mushroom**: This medicinal mushroom is known for its neuroprotective properties and has been shown to promote nerve growth factor (NGF), which supports axon regeneration and neural repair.
   - **Gotu Kola**: An adaptogenic herb that enhances blood circulation and is known to promote nerve regeneration and reduce oxidative stress in axons.
   - **Ginseng**: Supports cognitive function and enhances nerve regeneration, helping to protect axons and promote neural communication.
2. **Vitamins**:
   - **Vitamin B12**: Essential for the maintenance of myelin sheaths

around axons, vitamin B12 helps
prevent axonal degeneration and
supports overall nerve function.

- **Vitamin E**: Acts as a powerful
  antioxidant that protects axons
  from oxidative damage and
  supports healthy nerve cell
  membranes.
- **Vitamin D**: Promotes axonal
  growth and neuroplasticity by
  supporting the immune system
  and reducing inflammation in
  neural tissues.

3. **Minerals**:

- **Magnesium**: Supports the
  proper function of the nervous
  system and helps regulate the
  electrical activity within neurons,
  enhancing axon transmission.
- **Zinc**: Plays a role in synaptic
  transmission and is crucial for
  proper nerve function, including
  axonal health and the
  regeneration of nerve cells.
- **Copper**: Involved in the
  production of myelin, copper
  helps maintain the integrity of
  the axon and supports efficient
  signal conduction.

4. **Supplements**:
    - **Omega-3 Fatty Acids (DHA)**: DHA is crucial for maintaining the structure and function of the cell membranes in axons, promoting efficient signal transmission and axonal regeneration.
    - **Acetyl-L-Carnitine (ALCAR)**: Known for its neuroprotective properties, ALCAR enhances mitochondrial function in neurons and supports the regeneration of axons after injury.
    - **Alpha-Lipoic Acid (ALA)**: A potent antioxidant that helps protect axons from oxidative stress and supports healthy nerve function, particularly in cases of peripheral neuropathy.

These herbs, vitamins, minerals, and supplements work synergistically to protect, repair, and optimize the function of axons, ensuring that neural communication remains efficient and resilient.

Brain

The **brain** is the central organ of the human nervous system and is responsible for controlling all bodily functions, interpreting sensory information, and facilitating cognitive abilities such as thought, memory, and emotion. It is composed of approximately 86 billion neurons that communicate through trillions of synapses, making it one of the most complex systems known.

Structure of the Brain

The brain can be divided into several major regions, each with distinct functions:

1. **Cerebrum**: The largest part of the brain, responsible for higher cognitive functions such as reasoning, problem-solving, decision-making, voluntary movement, and sensory perception. It is divided into two hemispheres (left and right), each controlling the opposite side of the body.
   - **Frontal Lobe**: Involved in decision-making, planning, voluntary movement, and emotional regulation.

- **Parietal Lobe**: Processes sensory information such as touch, temperature, and pain.
  - **Temporal Lobe**: Associated with memory, auditory processing, and language comprehension.
  - **Occipital Lobe**: Responsible for visual processing.
2. **Cerebellum**: Located under the cerebrum, the cerebellum is responsible for coordinating voluntary movements, balance, posture, and motor learning.
3. **Brainstem**: The brainstem connects the brain to the spinal cord and controls vital life-sustaining functions such as heart rate, breathing, and blood pressure. It consists of:
   - **Midbrain**: Coordinates movement, particularly eye movement, and processes auditory and visual information.
   - **Pons**: Regulates breathing, sleep, and communication between different parts of the brain.
   - **Medulla Oblongata**: Controls autonomic functions such as heartbeat and respiration.

4. **Diencephalon**: Located between the cerebrum and the brainstem, the diencephalon includes structures that are crucial for sensory integration and hormonal regulation:
    - **Thalamus**: Acts as the brain's relay station, filtering and directing sensory information to the appropriate parts of the brain.
    - **Hypothalamus**: Regulates essential bodily functions such as hunger, thirst, sleep, and body temperature, and plays a key role in hormone release through its connection with the pituitary gland.
5. **Limbic System**: Often referred to as the "emotional brain," the limbic system regulates emotions, memory, and behavior. Key components include:
    - **Amygdala**: Processes emotions such as fear and pleasure.
    - **Hippocampus**: Essential for forming new memories and connecting emotions to them.
6. **Ventricles and Cerebrospinal Fluid (CSF)**: The brain has four interconnected cavities called ventricles that produce and circulate cerebrospinal

fluid. This fluid cushions the brain, removes waste products and delivers nutrients.

Function of the Brain

The brain is responsible for processing all incoming sensory information, sending out motor commands, regulating bodily functions, and supporting cognitive processes such as learning, memory, and problem-solving.

- **Sensory Processing**: The brain interprets sensory data (sight, sound, touch, taste, smell) from the body's sensory organs.
- **Motor Control**: The brain directs voluntary and involuntary movements through motor neurons.
- **Cognition**: Includes memory, attention, language, and reasoning.
- **Emotion**: The brain regulates mood, emotional responses, and behavioral impulses through the limbic system.
- **Homeostasis**: The brain maintains internal balance by regulating systems like temperature, hydration, and hormone production.

Herbs, Vitamins, Minerals, and Supplements (HVMS) for Brain Health

1. **Herbs**:
   - **Ginkgo Biloba**: Known for improving blood circulation to the brain, it enhances cognitive function and memory.
   - **Bacopa Monnieri**: A nootropic herb that supports memory, learning, and attention by promoting neuron communication and reducing anxiety.
   - **Ashwagandha**: An adaptogenic herb that helps reduce stress and improves cognitive function by modulating brain chemistry.
2. **Vitamins**:
   - **Vitamin B6, B9 (Folate), and B12**: These B vitamins support brain health by promoting neurotransmitter production and reducing levels of homocysteine, a compound linked to cognitive decline.
   - **Vitamin D**: Plays a role in cognitive function, mood

regulation, and protecting neurons from degeneration.

- **Vitamin E**: Acts as a powerful antioxidant, protecting brain cells from oxidative stress and supporting memory and cognitive performance.

3. **Minerals**:

   - **Magnesium**: Essential for nerve transmission and supporting synaptic plasticity, which is crucial for learning and memory.
   - **Zinc**: Plays a key role in modulating synaptic transmission and neuroplasticity, helping with cognitive and emotional processes.
   - **Iron**: Vital for oxygen transport to the brain, ensuring proper energy metabolism for cognitive function.

4. **Supplements**:

   - **Omega-3 Fatty Acids (DHA and EPA)**: Critical for brain structure and function, DHA supports neuronal membrane health, while EPA helps reduce inflammation that can lead to cognitive decline.

- **Phosphatidylserine**: A phospholipid that helps maintain cell membrane fluidity and enhances cognitive function, especially memory and attention.
- **Acetyl-L-Carnitine (ALCAR)**: Boosts brain energy metabolism and helps protect against neurodegeneration by improving mitochondrial function.

These nutrients and herbs help support brain function, protect neurons, and enhance cognitive performance, promoting overall brain health.

Cerebrum

The **cerebrum** is the largest and most developed part of the human brain, responsible for a wide array of complex functions such as reasoning, memory, sensory perception, voluntary movement, and language. It makes up the majority of the brain's volume and is divided into two hemispheres, which are further divided into four lobes with distinct functions.

Structure of the Cerebrum

1. **Hemispheres:**
   - **Left Hemisphere**: Primarily responsible for language, logical thinking, mathematical skills, and analytical processing. It controls the right side of the body.
   - **Right Hemisphere**: Associated with creativity, spatial awareness, artistic abilities, and holistic thinking. It controls the left side of the body.
2. Each hemisphere is connected by the **corpus callosum**, a thick band of nerve fibers that allows communication between them.
3. **Lobes of the Cerebrum:**

- **Frontal Lobe**: Located at the front of the brain, it is involved in voluntary movement, decision-making, problem-solving, and emotional regulation. The **prefrontal cortex**, found in this lobe, is crucial for higher cognitive functions such as planning and social behavior.
- **Parietal Lobe**: Positioned behind the frontal lobe, this region processes sensory information such as touch, temperature, and pain. It also helps with spatial orientation and navigation.
- **Temporal Lobe**: Located on the sides of the brain, this lobe is primarily responsible for auditory processing, language comprehension, and memory formation. The **hippocampus**, essential for memory, is found here.
- **Occipital Lobe**: Found at the back of the brain, the occipital lobe is responsible for visual processing, interpreting signals

from the eyes to create our perception of sight.

4. **Cerebral Cortex**:
   - The outer layer of the cerebrum is the **cerebral cortex**, composed of gray matter. This layer is densely packed with neurons and is involved in complex cognitive processes. The cortex is highly folded into **gyri** (ridges) and **sulci** (grooves) to increase surface area, allowing for more processing power.

5. **White Matter**:
   - Beneath the cortex lies **white matter**, made up of myelinated axons that facilitate communication between different areas of the cerebrum and other parts of the nervous system.

Functions of the Cerebrum

1. **Sensory Processing**: The cerebrum receives and interprets sensory information from all over the body. Each lobe specializes in processing different types of stimuli:
   - **Occipital Lobe** for vision
   - **Temporal Lobe** for hearing

- **Parietal Lobe** for touch, pain, and spatial awareness.

2. **Motor Control**: The **primary motor cortex** (located in the frontal lobe) initiates and controls voluntary movements, sending signals to the muscles to carry out actions.

3. **Cognitive Functions**: Higher-order thinking, including reasoning, judgment, attention, problem-solving, and planning, occurs mainly in the **prefrontal cortex** of the frontal lobe.

4. **Memory**: The **hippocampus**, located in the temporal lobe, plays a key role in converting short-term memories into long-term ones. The cerebrum is also involved in retrieving and manipulating stored information.

5. **Language**:
   - The **left hemisphere** houses regions like **Broca's area** (speech production) and **Wernicke's area** (language comprehension). Damage to these areas can result in speech or language difficulties.

6. **Emotion**: The **limbic system**, part of which is located within the cerebrum,

controls emotional responses, including fear, pleasure, and motivation.

7. **Consciousness and Awareness**: The cerebrum allows us to be aware of ourselves and our environment. It is central to consciousness, attention, and higher cognitive functions.

Importance of the Cerebrum

The cerebrum is crucial to what makes us human, controlling our thoughts, actions, and perceptions. From everyday activities like walking and talking to complex tasks like solving problems or creating art, the cerebrum is the command center that coordinates and integrates all these functions.

Herbs, Vitamins, Minerals, and Supplements (HVMS) for Cerebrum Health

1. **Herbs**:
   - **Ginkgo Biloba**: Enhances cerebral blood flow, improves memory, and supports cognitive functions.
   - **Rhodiola Rosea**: Known to reduce mental fatigue, improve

cognitive function, and boost brain resilience.

- **Gotu Kola**: Traditionally used to promote brain health, it may enhance memory and cognitive function while reducing anxiety.

2. **Vitamins**:
   - **Vitamin B12**: Supports nerve health and cognitive function by aiding in the production of myelin, the protective sheath around nerves.
   - **Vitamin B6**: Plays a role in neurotransmitter synthesis, which is crucial for brain communication.
   - **Vitamin C**: As an antioxidant, it protects the brain from oxidative damage and helps in the synthesis of neurotransmitters.

3. **Minerals**:
   - **Magnesium**: Helps in regulating neurotransmitters that are vital for learning and memory.
   - **Zinc**: Essential for neurotransmitter function and brain plasticity, which is key for learning and memory.

- ○ **Iron**: Vital for oxygen transport to the brain, necessary for energy production and cognitive function.
4. **Supplements**:
    - ○ **Omega-3 Fatty Acids (DHA and EPA)**: Critical for brain structure and function, particularly in the development and maintenance of healthy brain cells.
    - ○ **Phosphatidylserine**: Supports the structure of brain cells, enhances memory, and improves cognitive function.
    - ○ **Acetyl-L-Carnitine**: Aids in energy production in brain cells and supports mental clarity and focus.

These nutrients and herbs play essential roles in maintaining the health of the cerebrum, supporting its intricate functions, and protecting it from age-related decline.

Cerebellum

The **cerebellum** is a crucial part of the brain located at the back, beneath the cerebrum, and behind the brainstem. Often referred to as the "little brain" because of its distinct shape, the cerebellum is primarily responsible for coordinating movement, balance, posture, and fine motor skills. Though smaller in size compared to the cerebrum, it contains roughly half the neurons in the brain, emphasizing its role in processing complex neural signals.

Structure of the Cerebellum

The cerebellum is divided into two hemispheres and consists of three main layers:

1. **Outer Layer (Cerebellar Cortex):** Composed of gray matter, this layer is responsible for processing incoming motor and sensory signals.
2. **Inner Layer (White Matter):** Beneath the gray matter, this layer consists of nerve fibers (axons) that communicate with other parts of the brain.
3. **Deep Cerebellar Nuclei:** These are clusters of neurons deep within the white matter that relay the cerebellum's

output to other parts of the nervous system.

The cerebellum is divided into three main functional areas:

1. **Vestibulocerebellum**: Responsible for maintaining balance and eye movements, receiving input from the vestibular system of the inner ear.
2. **Spinocerebellum**: Controls posture and locomotion, integrating sensory feedback with motor commands for smooth, coordinated movement.
3. **Cerebrocerebellum**: Involved in planning, initiating voluntary movements, and fine-tuning motor actions.

Functions of the Cerebellum

1. **Coordination of Voluntary Movements:**
   - The cerebellum helps fine-tune voluntary movements, ensuring they are smooth and coordinated. It receives input from the motor cortex about intended movements and adjusts them

based on sensory feedback from the body.

2. **Balance and Posture**:
   - The cerebellum plays a central role in maintaining equilibrium. It continuously monitors sensory input from the body (such as from the inner ear and muscles) to make adjustments that help maintain balance and a stable posture.

3. **Motor Learning**:
   - The cerebellum is crucial for motor learning, such as learning to ride a bike or play a musical instrument. It stores learned motor skills and refines motor patterns over time through practice.

4. **Fine Motor Control**:
   - The cerebellum is responsible for the precision of fine motor tasks, such as writing, drawing, or playing an instrument, ensuring that movements are fluid and accurate.

5. **Cognitive and Emotional Roles**:
   - Though primarily involved in motor control, research has

shown that the cerebellum also contributes to certain cognitive functions like language and emotional regulation, supporting the brain's ability to manage thoughts and emotions.

6. **Error Detection and Correction**:
    - One of the cerebellum's most critical functions is detecting discrepancies between intended and actual movements and making real-time adjustments to correct errors, enabling smooth and precise motor actions.

Importance of the Cerebellum

The cerebellum ensures that movements are fluid, balanced, and precise. Damage to the cerebellum can result in a loss of coordination (ataxia), tremors, difficulty with balance, and impaired fine motor skills, significantly affecting day-to-day activities. While it does not initiate movement, it is indispensable for refining and correcting motions.

Herbs, Vitamins, Minerals, and Supplements (HVMS) for Cerebellum Health

1. **Herbs**:
   - **Bacopa Monnieri**: Supports cognitive function and motor learning by enhancing communication between neurons.
   - **Ashwagandha**: Known for its neuroprotective properties, it helps combat stress and supports brain health, including the cerebellum.
   - **Ginkgo Biloba**: Improves blood circulation to the brain, aiding the cerebellum's ability to receive oxygen and nutrients.
2. **Vitamins**:
   - **Vitamin E**: Acts as an antioxidant that protects brain cells, including those in the cerebellum, from oxidative stress.
   - **Vitamin B1 (Thiamine)**: Supports nervous system health and is crucial for maintaining motor coordination and cognitive function.

- **Vitamin D**: Plays a role in brain development and function, aiding in neuroplasticity, which is essential for motor learning.

3. **Minerals**:
   - **Magnesium**: Helps regulate nerve function and is important for motor control and muscle coordination.
   - **Calcium**: Vital for proper neurotransmission in the cerebellum, as it aids in the release of neurotransmitters essential for motor communication.
   - **Zinc**: Supports neuroplasticity and brain function, promoting motor learning and fine-tuning of movement.

4. **Supplements**:
   - **Omega-3 Fatty Acids**: Essential for brain health, they support neuronal communication and protect against neurodegeneration.
   - **Coenzyme Q10 (CoQ10)**: Boosts energy production in brain cells and acts as an

antioxidant, protecting the cerebellum from damage.
- **Alpha-Lipoic Acid**: A potent antioxidant that protects neurons in the cerebellum from oxidative stress and inflammation.

By nourishing the cerebellum through proper nutrition, herbs, and supplements, you can enhance motor coordination, balance, and fine motor skills, ensuring your movements remain smooth and precise throughout life.

Brainstem

The **brainstem** is one of the most vital structures in the brain, located at the base, where it connects the brain to the spinal cord. It is responsible for controlling many automatic, life-sustaining functions such as breathing, heart rate, and blood pressure. The brainstem also acts as a relay center, transmitting signals between the brain and the rest of the body.

Structure of the Brainstem

The brainstem is divided into three main parts:

1. **Midbrain (Mesencephalon):**
   - The uppermost part of the brainstem, the midbrain is involved in regulating movement, particularly in response to visual and auditory stimuli. It also plays a role in the control of eye movements and pupil dilation.
2. **Pons:**
   - The pons are located below the midbrain and serve as a bridge between various parts of the brain, including the cerebellum and the cerebral cortex. It plays a

crucial role in regulating breathing, facial sensations, and movement, as well as sleep cycles.

3. **Medulla Oblongata**:
    - The lowest part of the brainstem, the medulla oblongata controls essential involuntary functions like heart rate, blood pressure, and reflexes such as coughing, sneezing, and swallowing. It is also responsible for regulating respiration.

Functions of the Brainstem

1. **Autonomic Control**:
    - The brainstem is responsible for regulating involuntary functions that keep the body alive, such as heart rate, blood pressure, breathing, and digestion.
2. **Sensory and Motor Pathways**:
    - The brainstem acts as a conduit for sensory and motor information traveling between the brain and the spinal cord. It helps coordinate and refine these signals for proper body movement and sensation.
3. **Reflexes**:

- The brainstem controls many reflex actions, such as swallowing, vomiting, coughing, and sneezing, which are critical for protecting the body from harm.

4. **Sleep and Arousal**:
   - The brainstem plays a crucial role in regulating sleep-wake cycles and maintaining consciousness. It helps the body switch between states of alertness and rest.

5. **Cranial Nerve Control**:
   - The brainstem houses the nuclei of several cranial nerves, which control facial expressions, eye movement, hearing, balance, and swallowing.

6. **Coordination of Movements**:
   - The brainstem works in tandem with the cerebellum to help coordinate smooth, controlled movements, particularly those involved in posture and balance.

Importance of the Brainstem

The brainstem is vital for survival, as it controls many of the body's critical functions. Damage to the brainstem can result in severe consequences, including impaired breathing, loss of consciousness, or even death. Conditions like strokes, tumors, or traumatic injuries affecting the brainstem are often life-threatening and require immediate medical attention.

Herbs, Vitamins, Minerals, and Supplements (HVMS) for Brainstem Health

1. **Herbs**:
   - **Rhodiola Rosea**: Helps reduce fatigue and enhance brain function, supporting the brainstem's role in regulating energy levels and stress responses.
   - **Ginseng**: Known for its neuroprotective properties, ginseng improves mental clarity and supports the brainstem's role in regulating cognition and alertness.
   - **Gotu Kola**: Enhances blood flow to the brain, which can help the brainstem perform its vital functions more efficiently.
2. **Vitamins**:

- **Vitamin B6 (Pyridoxine)**: Essential for neurotransmitter production, which helps the brainstem regulate many autonomic and reflexive functions.
- **Vitamin B12**: Vital for maintaining the health of nerve cells, ensuring proper signal transmission between the brainstem and the rest of the body.
- **Vitamin C**: Acts as a powerful antioxidant that protects the brainstem from oxidative stress and inflammation.

3. **Minerals**:
    - **Magnesium**: Regulates nerve transmission and muscle contraction, which is crucial for the brainstem's role in controlling autonomic functions like breathing and heartbeat.
    - **Selenium**: A powerful antioxidant that protects brainstem cells from oxidative damage and supports overall brain health.

- o **Iron**: Essential for oxygen transport, iron helps ensure that the brainstem receives adequate oxygen to perform its critical functions.
4. **Supplements**:
   - o **Phosphatidylserine**: Supports cognitive function and protects nerve cells in the brainstem, helping maintain communication between the brain and the body.
   - o **L-Theanine**: Promotes relaxation and alertness by regulating neurotransmitters, supporting the brainstem's role in sleep and wakefulness.
   - o **Acetyl-L-Carnitine**: Enhances brain function and supports energy production in brainstem cells, which is crucial for maintaining vital functions.

Supporting the brainstem through proper nutrition and supplementation can help protect this critical part of the brain and ensure that it continues to regulate the body's essential functions effectively.

Spinal Cord

The **spinal cord** is a long, cylindrical bundle of nerve fibers that extends from the brainstem (specifically the medulla oblongata) down through the vertebral column, ending around the lower back in the lumbar region. It serves as the main pathway for transmitting information between the brain and the rest of the body. The spinal cord plays a crucial role in motor control, sensory perception, and reflex actions, and it acts as a highway for the brain's instructions to muscles and organs.

Structure of the Spinal Cord

The spinal cord is divided into different segments that correspond to different regions of the body. These segments include:

1. **Cervical Region (C1-C8)**:
    - The uppermost section, located in the neck, controls signals to the head, neck, diaphragm, arms, and hands.
2. **Thoracic Region (T1-T12)**:
    - Located in the upper back, this region controls signals to the chest, back muscles, and parts of the abdomen.

3. **Lumbar Region (L1-L5)**:
    - Located in the lower back, it controls signals to the hips, lower abdomen, and legs.
4. **Sacral Region (S1-S5)**:
    - This region controls signals to the pelvis, buttocks, genitals, and lower legs and feet.
5. **Coccygeal Region (1 segment)**:
    - The lowest part of the spinal cord is located near the coccyx or tailbone.

Gray Matter vs. White Matter

The spinal cord is composed of two main types of tissue:

- **Gray Matter**: Located in the center of the spinal cord, gray matter is shaped like a butterfly or the letter "H" in cross-sections. It contains neuron cell bodies and is responsible for processing and integrating information.
- **White Matter**: Surrounding the gray matter, white matter consists of myelinated nerve fibers (axons) that form communication highways for signals to travel between the brain and the body.

Functions of the Spinal Cord

1. **Transmission of Signals**:
   - The spinal cord serves as the primary conduit for signals traveling between the brain and the peripheral nervous system. Motor signals from the brain to muscles are transmitted via the spinal cord, while sensory information from the body travels back up to the brain for processing.
2. **Reflex Actions**:
   - The spinal cord is responsible for processing reflexes, which are automatic, rapid responses to stimuli that don't require brain involvement. For instance, if you touch something hot, your spinal cord will initiate a reflexive withdrawal of your hand without waiting for your brain to process the sensation.
3. **Motor Control**:
   - The spinal cord transmits motor commands from the brain to muscles, enabling movement and coordination. It also ensures that muscles work in a smooth,

coordinated fashion, facilitating activities like walking and running.

4. **Sensory Information Processing**:
   - The spinal cord carries sensory signals (such as touch, pressure, pain, and temperature) from different parts of the body to the brain, enabling conscious perception and response to external stimuli.

5. **Autonomic Functions**:
   - Certain aspects of the autonomic nervous system, such as bladder control and bowel movements, are regulated through the spinal cord.

Spinal Nerves

Thirty-one pairs of **spinal nerves** extend from the spinal cord to various parts of the body, each carrying motor, sensory, and autonomic signals. These nerves emerge from the spinal cord at regular intervals and are named according to the region they come from (e.g., cervical, thoracic, lumbar, sacral).

Clinical Significance

Injuries to the spinal cord can result in partial or complete paralysis, depending on the severity and location of the damage. For example:

- **Cervical injuries** may result in quadriplegia (paralysis of all four limbs).
- **Thoracic or lumbar injuries** may result in paraplegia (paralysis of the lower limbs).

Spinal cord injuries are often permanent because nerve fibers in the spinal cord do not easily regenerate. Conditions like herniated discs, spinal stenosis, and multiple sclerosis can also affect spinal cord function.

Herbs, Vitamins, Minerals, and Supplements (HVMS) for Spinal Cord Health

1. **Herbs**:
    - **Turmeric (Curcumin)**: Known for its anti-inflammatory properties, turmeric can help reduce inflammation around the spinal cord and protect it from oxidative stress.
    - **Ashwagandha**: This adaptogenic herb supports nerve

function and helps the body cope with stress, which can benefit spinal cord health and recovery from injury.

- **Boswellia Serrata**: Another potent anti-inflammatory herb, Boswellia helps reduce inflammation and can support spinal cord function, especially in cases of chronic pain or injury.

2. **Vitamins**:

- **Vitamin B12**: Crucial for maintaining the health of the myelin sheath that protects nerve fibers, including those in the spinal cord. A deficiency in B12 can lead to nerve damage and impaired spinal cord function.
- **Vitamin D**: Supports bone health and helps reduce the risk of spinal cord injury by keeping the vertebrae strong. It also aids in reducing inflammation.
- **Vitamin C**: Acts as an antioxidant and helps in collagen formation, which is vital for spinal cord health, especially after injury.

3. **Minerals**:

- **Magnesium**: Known for its role in muscle relaxation and nerve function, magnesium helps support spinal cord function and can reduce muscle spasms associated with nerve injuries.
- **Calcium**: Essential for maintaining the strength of the vertebrae that protect the spinal cord. A healthy supply of calcium is necessary to prevent fractures or bone degradation.
- **Zinc**: Promotes the repair of damaged tissues and supports overall nervous system function, which is crucial for the spinal cord.

4. **Supplements**:
   - **Omega-3 Fatty Acids**: These have neuroprotective properties and can help regenerate nerve cells, including those in the spinal cord. Omega-3s also reduce inflammation and improve overall nerve health.
   - **N-Acetyl Cysteine (NAC)**: A potent antioxidant, NAC can help protect spinal cord neurons from

oxidative damage and promote healing in cases of injury.
  - **Glucosamine and Chondroitin**: These supplements support spinal health by promoting the repair and maintenance of the cartilage and connective tissues around the spinal cord, reducing pressure on the nerves.

Ensuring the spinal cord receives adequate nutritional support through these herbs, vitamins, minerals, and supplements can promote nerve function, reduce inflammation, and support the overall health and resilience of the spinal cord.

Peripheral Nerves

Peripheral nerves are the vast network of nerves that extend beyond the brain and spinal cord, forming the **Peripheral Nervous System (PNS)**. These nerves connect the central nervous system (CNS) to the limbs and organs, enabling communication between the brain, spinal cord, and the rest of the body. Peripheral nerves play a critical role in transmitting sensory information to the CNS and conveying motor commands to muscles and organs.

Structure and Function

Each peripheral nerve is made up of bundles of nerve fibers (axons), which are covered by layers of connective tissue:

1. **Epineurium**: The outermost layer that encloses the entire nerve.
2. **Perineurium**: Surrounds bundles (fascicles) of nerve fibers within the nerve.
3. **Endoneurium**: The innermost layer that surrounds individual axons and their myelin sheath.

There are three main types of peripheral nerves, each serving distinct functions:

1. **Sensory (Afferent) Nerves**: These carry signals from sensory receptors in the skin, muscles, and organs to the brain and spinal cord. They transmit information such as pain, temperature, touch, and proprioception (body position awareness).
2. **Motor (Efferent) Nerves**: These carry signals from the CNS to muscles, allowing voluntary and involuntary movements. Motor nerves control muscle contractions and glandular secretions.
3. **Autonomic Nerves**: Part of the autonomic nervous system (ANS), these nerves regulate involuntary functions such as heart rate, digestion, and respiratory rate. They are further divided into:
    - **Sympathetic Nerves**: Responsible for the "fight or flight" response.
    - **Parasympathetic Nerves**: Control the "rest and digest" functions.

Peripheral Nerve Function and Communication

Peripheral nerves facilitate communication between the CNS and the rest of the body through **synaptic transmission**, where electrical impulses travel along axons and trigger neurotransmitter release at synapses. This process is essential for motor coordination, sensory perception, and maintaining homeostasis.

Damage to Peripheral Nerves

Peripheral nerves can be damaged by a variety of factors, leading to **peripheral neuropathy**. Common causes include:

- **Physical Trauma**: Injuries like cuts, compressions, or fractures can sever or damage peripheral nerves.
- **Diabetes**: High blood sugar levels can damage nerves, particularly in the hands and feet, leading to diabetic neuropathy.
- **Infections**: Certain infections, like Lyme disease or shingles, can damage peripheral nerves.
- **Autoimmune Diseases**: Conditions like Guillain-Barré syndrome or lupus can result in nerve damage.

Symptoms of peripheral nerve damage include numbness, tingling, muscle weakness, burning sensations, and difficulty coordinating movements.

Herbs, Vitamins, Minerals, and Supplements (HVMS) for Peripheral Nerve Health

1. **Herbs**:
   - **St. John's Wort**: Known for its nerve-soothing properties, St. John's Wort may help reduce nerve pain and inflammation associated with peripheral neuropathy.
   - **Skullcap**: This herb has neuroprotective properties and can help calm nerve irritation, reducing discomfort from nerve damage.
   - **Ginkgo Biloba**: Improves blood circulation, especially to peripheral nerves, which can enhance nerve regeneration and function.
2. **Vitamins**:
   - **Vitamin B12**: Critical for maintaining nerve health,

especially for myelin sheath repair, which protects nerve fibers. B12 deficiency is a common cause of peripheral neuropathy.

- **Vitamin B6**: Supports neurotransmitter synthesis and nerve function, but should be taken in moderation since too much B6 can cause nerve damage.
- **Vitamin E**: Acts as a powerful antioxidant that protects nerves from oxidative stress and promotes healing.

3. **Minerals**:
- **Magnesium**: Helps relax muscles and supports normal nerve function. It is beneficial for managing nerve-related pain and spasms.
- **Zinc**: Plays a role in nerve repair and regeneration, particularly after injury.
- **Calcium**: Necessary for proper nerve signaling and muscle function. A lack of calcium can lead to muscle cramps and spasms.

4. **Supplements**:
    - **Alpha-Lipoic Acid**: A potent antioxidant that can reduce inflammation and improve nerve function, particularly in people with diabetic neuropathy.
    - **Acetyl-L-Carnitine**: Helps regenerate nerve cells and supports mitochondrial energy production in nerves, promoting faster healing after damage.
    - **Omega-3 Fatty Acids**: These essential fats provide anti-inflammatory benefits and support nerve regeneration, particularly in cases of peripheral nerve injuries.

By nourishing the peripheral nerves with a combination of herbs, vitamins, minerals, and supplements, it is possible to promote nerve repair, reduce inflammation, and support overall nervous system health. This can aid in preventing or managing conditions like neuropathy and restoring healthy nerve function.

Somatic Nervous System (SNS)

The **Somatic Nervous System (SNS)** is a critical part of the **Peripheral Nervous System (PNS)** that is responsible for voluntary control of body movements. It connects the **central nervous system (CNS)**—the brain and spinal cord—with the skeletal muscles, allowing for conscious and intentional actions. The SNS also transmits sensory information from the skin, muscles, and sensory organs back to the CNS, enabling perception of the external environment.

Structure and Components

The somatic nervous system has two main components:

1. **Sensory (Afferent) Pathways**:
   - These pathways carry sensory signals from the external environment and body (such as touch, pain, temperature, and body position) to the CNS. Sensory receptors in the skin, muscles, and joints detect changes and send information to the brain and spinal cord for processing.

2. **Motor (Efferent) Pathways**:
   - These pathways transmit motor commands from the CNS to the skeletal muscles, controlling voluntary movement. This involves the transmission of impulses from motor neurons in the spinal cord or brain to specific muscle fibers, initiating contraction and movement.

Key Functions of the SNS

- **Voluntary Movements**: The SNS governs all voluntary actions, such as walking, talking, lifting objects, and any intentional use of skeletal muscles. Motor neurons are activated when the brain sends signals to execute these movements.
- **Reflex Arcs**: Although the SNS is generally involved in voluntary control, it also governs reflex actions, which occur automatically without conscious thought. Reflex arcs, like the knee-jerk response, allow the body to react quickly to stimuli, protecting it from harm.
- **Sensory Feedback**: The SNS provides feedback from the external environment through sensory receptors. This sensory

information is crucial for maintaining balance, coordination, and awareness of body position (proprioception).

Neural Pathways and Communication

The SNS primarily communicates via **somatic motor neurons** located in the spinal cord and brainstem. These neurons extend through peripheral nerves to reach muscle fibers. When a motor neuron receives a signal from the CNS, it releases the neurotransmitter **acetylcholine** at the **neuromuscular junction**, causing the muscle to contract.

In sensory pathways, **sensory neurons** detect external stimuli and convert them into electrical impulses that travel through the peripheral nerves to the CNS. This feedback loop helps the brain process sensations like touch, pressure, and pain, facilitating interaction with the environment.

Disorders of the Somatic Nervous System

Several conditions can affect the function of the SNS, particularly when motor neurons or sensory pathways are damaged. These include:

- **Neuromuscular Disorders**: Diseases like amyotrophic lateral sclerosis (ALS) or muscular dystrophy can impair voluntary muscle control, leading to weakness, paralysis, or muscle atrophy.

- **Peripheral Neuropathy**: Damage to sensory nerves in the SNS can cause numbness, tingling, or pain, particularly in the hands and feet, often due to diabetes or trauma.
- **Spinal Cord Injuries**: Damage to the spinal cord can sever communication between the brain and peripheral nerves, leading to loss of motor control and sensation below the injury site.

Herbs, Vitamins, Minerals, and Supplements (HVMS) for Somatic Nervous System Health

1. **Herbs**:
   - **Ashwagandha**: Known for its neuroprotective effects, ashwagandha may help reduce inflammation in nerves and support overall nervous system function.
   - **Bacopa Monnieri**: This herb enhances cognitive function and protects nerve cells from

oxidative damage, which is beneficial for the somatic nervous system.

- o **Gotu Kola**: A powerful herb for nerve regeneration and repair, Gotu Kola improves circulation and promotes healing of nerve tissues.

2. **Vitamins**:

- o **Vitamin B12**: Essential for the maintenance and repair of the myelin sheath around nerves, Vitamin B12 supports motor neuron function and prevents nerve damage.
- o **Vitamin D**: Helps regulate the nervous system, particularly in maintaining healthy nerve signaling and muscle function.
- o **Vitamin C**: An antioxidant that protects neurons from oxidative stress and assists in collagen production, crucial for tissue repair in nerves.

3. **Minerals**:

- o **Magnesium**: A key mineral for nerve transmission and muscle relaxation, magnesium helps prevent muscle cramps and supports nerve health.

- **Potassium**: Vital for nerve impulse transmission, potassium maintains proper communication between nerves and muscles.
- **Calcium**: Plays a crucial role in neuromuscular junction function, assisting in the release of neurotransmitters that trigger muscle contractions.

4. **Supplements**:
- **N-Acetyl Cysteine (NAC)**: An antioxidant that helps protect neurons from oxidative stress and enhances recovery in the nervous system.
- **Coenzyme Q10 (CoQ10)**: Supports mitochondrial function in nerve cells, ensuring they have the energy needed to transmit signals effectively.
- **Acetyl-L-Carnitine**: Promotes nerve regeneration and improves nerve cell function, aiding in the repair of damaged somatic nerves.

By combining a nutrient-rich diet with targeted supplements and herbs, you can help maintain the health of your somatic nervous system, ensuring that your body remains responsive, coordinated, and resilient in the face of both voluntary movements and reflex actions.

Autonomic Nervous System (ANS)

The **Autonomic Nervous System (ANS)** is a vital component of the **Peripheral Nervous System (PNS)** responsible for controlling involuntary bodily functions. Unlike the **Somatic Nervous System (SNS)**, which manages voluntary muscle movements, the ANS operates automatically, regulating essential functions such as heart rate, digestion, respiratory rate, and blood pressure. It ensures that the body's internal environment remains stable and responds appropriately to external changes, without conscious effort.

Structure and Divisions

The ANS is divided into two primary branches:

1. **Sympathetic Nervous System (SNS)**:
    - Often referred to as the "fight or flight" system, the **sympathetic division** prepares the body for stressful or emergency situations. It accelerates processes such as heart rate and respiration while inhibiting non-essential activities like digestion.

2. **Parasympathetic Nervous System (PNS)**:
    - ○ Known as the "rest and digest" system, the **parasympathetic division** works to conserve energy by slowing down bodily processes when the body is at rest. It promotes activities like digestion and recovery, lowering the heart rate and encouraging relaxation.

These two divisions work in tandem to maintain **homeostasis**, adjusting bodily functions based on external or internal stimuli.

Functions of the Autonomic Nervous System

The ANS controls a wide range of involuntary processes, including:

- **Heart Rate**: The ANS adjusts the rate and strength of heart contractions, balancing the sympathetic and parasympathetic signals to maintain cardiovascular health.
- **Respiratory Rate**: Increases or decreases the rate of breathing according to oxygen demands, particularly during exercise or at rest.

- **Digestive Processes**: Regulates smooth muscle contraction in the gastrointestinal tract, controls the release of digestive enzymes, and monitors nutrient absorption.
- **Pupil Dilation**: Controls the constriction or dilation of the pupils in response to light and other stimuli.
- **Blood Pressure**: Adjusts blood vessel dilation and contraction to regulate blood pressure, ensuring that vital organs receive sufficient blood flow.
- **Body Temperature Regulation**: Manages processes such as sweating and blood flow to the skin, keeping the body's temperature within an optimal range.
- **Glandular Secretions**: Regulates the function of sweat glands, salivary glands, and adrenal glands, coordinating responses to stress and relaxation.

Autonomic Pathways

The ANS communicates through a two-neuron system consisting of **preganglionic** and **postganglionic neurons**:

- **Preganglionic Neurons**: Originate in the CNS and extend to an autonomic

ganglion where they synapse with postganglionic neurons.
- **Postganglionic Neurons**: Extend from the ganglia to the target organs, where they transmit signals to initiate appropriate responses in muscles, glands, or organs.

Neurotransmitters play a critical role in ANS signaling. The **sympathetic division** primarily uses **norepinephrine** (adrenaline) to activate target organs, while the **parasympathetic division** relies on **acetylcholine** to promote calming and restorative functions.

Disorders of the ANS

Dysfunction in the ANS can lead to a variety of disorders, affecting both the sympathetic and parasympathetic systems. Some common ANS disorders include:

- **Dysautonomia**: A general term for dysfunction in the autonomic nervous system, leading to problems with blood pressure regulation, heart rate, digestion, and other automatic processes.

- **Postural Orthostatic Tachycardia Syndrome (POTS)**: A condition in which the body cannot properly regulate blood flow and blood pressure, causing symptoms like dizziness and fainting upon standing.
- **Autonomic Neuropathy**: Damage to the autonomic nerves, often caused by diabetes, leading to complications in heart rate, blood pressure, and digestion.

Herbs, Vitamins, Minerals, and Supplements (HVMS) for Autonomic Nervous System Health

1. **Herbs:**
   - **Rhodiola Rosea**: An adaptogen that helps balance the stress response by modulating the activity of the sympathetic nervous system, reducing anxiety and fatigue.
   - **Holy Basil (Tulsi)**: Promotes relaxation and helps to regulate the body's stress response, supporting the parasympathetic nervous system.

- **Valerian Root**: Known for its calming effects, valerian root helps ease tension and anxiety, supporting the parasympathetic system for better relaxation and sleep.

2. **Vitamins**:
   - **Vitamin B Complex**: Essential for nervous system health, particularly the regulation of neurotransmitter production that influences autonomic function.
   - **Vitamin D**: Supports nerve function and immune health, helping to regulate responses controlled by the autonomic nervous system.
   - **Vitamin E**: An antioxidant that helps protect the nerves from oxidative damage, promoting healthy autonomic nerve function.

3. **Minerals**:
   - **Magnesium**: Critical for calming the nervous system and preventing overactivity of the sympathetic system, magnesium supports relaxation and muscle function.

- o **Potassium**: Plays an important role in nerve transmission and muscle contraction, supporting the proper functioning of both the sympathetic and parasympathetic systems.
  - o **Zinc**: Supports immune health and nerve function, aiding in the regulation of autonomic responses.
4. **Supplements**:
  - o **L-Theanine**: Found in green tea, this amino acid promotes relaxation without drowsiness, balancing the autonomic nervous system by enhancing parasympathetic activity.
  - o **Phosphatidylserine**: Helps reduce the effects of stress on the body, supporting the sympathetic system during heightened stress response.
  - o **Omega-3 Fatty Acids**: Promotes nerve health and reduces inflammation, supporting optimal autonomic function, particularly in maintaining heart rate and blood pressure.

Incorporating these herbs, vitamins, minerals, and supplements into your lifestyle can help maintain the balance and health of the autonomic nervous system, fostering a state of calm, resilience, and overall wellness.

Sympathetic Nervous System (SNS)

The **Sympathetic Nervous System (SNS)** is one of the two primary divisions of the **Autonomic Nervous System (ANS)** and is responsible for the body's "fight or flight" response. It prepares the body to react to stressful or dangerous situations by rapidly mobilizing resources to cope with physical and psychological stressors. When activated, the SNS increases heart rate, redirects blood to essential organs and muscles, dilates the airways, and inhibits non-essential functions like digestion, allowing the body to focus on immediate survival.

Key Functions of the Sympathetic Nervous System

- **Heart Rate and Blood Pressure**: The SNS stimulates the heart to beat faster and stronger, increasing blood pressure to ensure that oxygen and nutrients reach muscles and vital organs.
- **Respiratory System**: Airways dilate to increase airflow to the lungs, providing more oxygen to the body during times of stress or exertion.
- **Energy Mobilization**: The SNS triggers the release of glucose (sugar) from energy stores like the liver to

provide muscles with immediate energy for action.

- **Pupil Dilation**: The SNS dilates the pupils, allowing more light to enter the eyes and improving vision in low-light conditions.
- **Blood Flow Redistribution**: Blood is redirected away from the digestive tract and skin, and towards skeletal muscles, heart, and brain to prioritize their function during emergencies.
- **Sweating**: The SNS activates sweat glands to help regulate body temperature during periods of stress or physical exertion.
- **Inhibition of Digestive Functions**: Digestive processes slow down or stop, conserving energy for the body's immediate response to a perceived threat.

Pathways and Neurotransmitters

The SNS communicates through a complex pathway of neurons. **Preganglionic neurons** arise from the thoracic and lumbar regions of the spinal cord and extend to **sympathetic ganglia**, where they synapse with **postganglionic neurons**. These postganglionic neurons then send signals to target organs, such as the heart, lungs, and muscles.

The primary neurotransmitters used by the SNS include:

- **Norepinephrine (Noradrenaline)**: This is the main neurotransmitter released by postganglionic sympathetic neurons to activate the target tissues and organs.
- **Epinephrine (Adrenaline)**: Released by the adrenal glands, epinephrine amplifies the effects of the SNS, particularly during intense stress.

These neurotransmitters bind to adrenergic receptors on target organs to initiate the "fight or flight" response.

Health Implications of SNS Activation

While the sympathetic response is essential for survival, chronic or excessive activation of the SNS can lead to health problems, including:

- **Hypertension (High Blood Pressure)**: Constant SNS stimulation can keep blood pressure elevated, leading to cardiovascular problems.

- **Anxiety and Stress**: Prolonged SNS activation contributes to chronic stress and anxiety disorders, as the body remains in a heightened state of alertness.
- **Gastrointestinal Issues**: Reduced blood flow to the digestive organs over time can impair digestion and lead to issues like irritable bowel syndrome (IBS).
- **Insomnia**: Overactivation of the SNS can disrupt sleep patterns, leading to insomnia and other sleep disorders.

Herbs, Vitamins, Minerals, and Supplements (HVMS) for Sympathetic Nervous System Health

1. **Herbs**:
   - **Ashwagandha**: An adaptogen that helps modulate the body's stress response by balancing the overactivity of the SNS, reducing cortisol levels and anxiety.
   - **Siberian Ginseng**: Boosts energy and endurance, supporting the body during

stress, while also helping regulate SNS activity.

- ○ **Passionflower**: Has calming properties, helping to reduce SNS activation and promote relaxation.

2. **Vitamins**:
   - ○ **Vitamin C**: Supports adrenal function and reduces the production of stress hormones, helping to moderate the effects of SNS activation.
   - ○ **B-Complex Vitamins**: Particularly B5 (pantothenic acid) and B6 (pyridoxine), these are crucial for adrenal health and the synthesis of neurotransmitters like norepinephrine.
   - ○ **Vitamin D**: Low levels of vitamin D have been linked to stress and anxiety, as it plays a role in regulating mood and SNS activity.

3. **Minerals**:
   - ○ **Magnesium**: Helps relax the muscles and nervous system, countering excessive SNS stimulation by promoting parasympathetic activity.

- **Potassium**: Essential for proper nerve function and the regulation of heart rate and blood pressure, helping balance the SNS response.
  - **Calcium**: Important for neurotransmitter release and nerve signal transmission, ensuring balanced nervous system function.
4. **Supplements**:
  - **Phosphatidylserine**: A phospholipid that helps regulate cortisol levels and reduce the impact of chronic SNS activation, promoting a balanced stress response.
  - **Omega-3 Fatty Acids**: Known to reduce inflammation and improve brain function, omega-3s help modulate stress and sympathetic activity.
  - **L-Theanine**: Found in green tea, this amino acid promotes relaxation without sedation, helping to moderate SNS overactivity and reduce stress-related symptoms.

By incorporating these natural elements into your daily regimen, you can support the regulation of your sympathetic nervous system, reducing chronic stress and promoting a balanced "fight or flight" response when truly needed.

Parasympathetic Nervous System (PNS)

The **Parasympathetic Nervous System (PNS)** is the second major division of the **Autonomic Nervous System (ANS)**, often referred to as the "rest and digest" system. Its primary role is to conserve energy and promote the body's maintenance activities, particularly during periods of rest. The PNS counteracts the excitatory actions of the **Sympathetic Nervous System (SNS)** by slowing the heart rate, promoting digestion, and facilitating recovery processes. While the SNS prepares the body for immediate action, the PNS focuses on long-term stability and homeostasis.

Key Functions of the Parasympathetic Nervous System

- **Heart Rate and Blood Pressure**: The PNS slows the heart rate and reduces blood pressure, allowing the body to conserve energy and maintain a calm state.
- **Digestive System**: It stimulates digestion by promoting the secretion of saliva, gastric juices, and digestive enzymes, increasing blood flow to the

stomach and intestines, and enhancing peristalsis (the movement of food through the digestive tract).

- **Respiratory System**: The PNS constricts the airways when the body is at rest, regulating breathing and optimizing oxygen use during non-stressful situations.
- **Energy Conservation**: By reducing metabolic activity, the PNS helps conserve energy and directs it toward the body's healing and recovery processes.
- **Pupil Constriction**: The PNS contracts the pupils, reducing light intake and supporting restful states.
- **Urinary and Reproductive Functions**: It promotes bladder control, encouraging urination, and supports reproductive functions such as sexual arousal.

Pathways and Neurotransmitters

The PNS is mediated by **preganglionic neurons** originating from the brainstem and sacral regions of the spinal cord. These neurons synapse with **postganglionic neurons** near the target organs, allowing for localized and specific control over organs like the heart, lungs, and digestive system.

The primary neurotransmitter involved in parasympathetic activity is **acetylcholine**. It binds to **muscarinic receptors** on the target organs, initiating the "rest and digest" processes.

The Vagus Nerve

A crucial component of the PNS is the **vagus nerve (cranial nerve X)**. It is the longest cranial nerve and serves as the primary channel through which the PNS communicates with most internal organs, including the heart, lungs, liver, and digestive tract. Vagal tone, or the health of the vagus nerve, plays a vital role in regulating stress, emotional health, and overall physiological balance.

Health Implications of PNS Activation

Proper activation of the parasympathetic nervous system is essential for maintaining health and preventing stress-related disorders. Prolonged suppression of the PNS, usually caused by chronic SNS activation, can lead to health issues such as:

- **Chronic Stress and Anxiety**: Without regular activation of the PNS, the body remains in a heightened state of alertness, leading to constant stress and anxiety.
- **Digestive Disorders**: Insufficient parasympathetic activity can impair digestion, leading to conditions such as constipation, indigestion, and irritable bowel syndrome (IBS).
- **Heart Problems**: Low parasympathetic tone is associated with an increased risk of cardiovascular disease, as the PNS plays a crucial role in maintaining healthy heart function.
- **Weakened Immune System**: The PNS supports immune function, and when its activity is diminished, the body becomes more susceptible to infections and diseases.

The Balance Between SNS and PNS

A healthy autonomic nervous system requires a delicate balance between the SNS and PNS. While the SNS prepares the body for action, the PNS allows for recovery and restoration. Chronic stress, overstimulation, or trauma can disrupt this balance, leading to physical and mental health problems. Practices such as meditation, deep breathing, yoga, and mindfulness help restore the parasympathetic response, promoting relaxation and healing.

Herbs, Vitamins, Minerals, and Supplements (HVMS) for Parasympathetic Nervous System Health

1. **Herbs**:
   - **Chamomile**: Known for its calming effects, chamomile supports parasympathetic activity by reducing anxiety and promoting relaxation.
   - **Valerian Root**: A natural sedative, valerian root helps soothe the nervous system, enhancing the "rest and digest" response.
   - **Lemon Balm**: This herb promotes calmness and reduces stress, encouraging PNS activation and supporting digestive function.
2. **Vitamins**:
   - **Vitamin B1 (Thiamine)**: Helps maintain healthy nervous system function and supports

neurotransmitter balance in the parasympathetic pathways.

- **Vitamin B12**: Supports nerve health and helps regulate autonomic nervous system functions, including parasympathetic responses.
- **Folate (Vitamin B9)**: Important for neurological function, folate helps support a healthy nervous system and balanced neurotransmitter production.

3. **Minerals**:

- **Magnesium**: Plays a crucial role in calming the nervous system, reducing tension, and promoting parasympathetic activity. It helps lower heart rate and relax muscles.
- **Zinc**: Essential for maintaining proper nervous system function, zinc helps regulate neurotransmitter release and supports parasympathetic activity.
- **Calcium**: Supports the release of acetylcholine, the primary

neurotransmitter used by the parasympathetic nervous system.

4. **Supplements**:
    - **GABA (Gamma-Aminobutyric Acid)**: A neurotransmitter that promotes relaxation and reduces neuronal excitability, supporting the parasympathetic response.
    - **5-HTP (5-Hydroxytryptophan)**: Helps increase serotonin levels in the brain, promoting calmness and improving vagal tone, which supports the parasympathetic nervous system.
    - **L-Theanine**: Found in green tea, this amino acid enhances relaxation and helps balance autonomic nervous system activity, promoting parasympathetic dominance.

By nurturing the parasympathetic nervous system through a balanced lifestyle and natural supplementation, you can foster calm, enhance digestion, and support the body's natural healing and recovery processes.

Nerve Impulse

A **nerve impulse**, also known as an **action potential**, is the electrical signal transmitted along neurons (nerve cells) to relay information throughout the body. This fundamental process allows the nervous system to communicate with muscles, organs, and other systems, controlling everything from voluntary movements to automatic functions like breathing and heart rate. The nerve impulse is generated through the coordinated action of ions moving across the neuronal membrane, resulting in the propagation of an electrical signal.

How Nerve Impulses Work: The Action Potential

The action potential involves a series of electrical and chemical changes that occur in the neuron's membrane. This process can be broken down into several key steps:

1. **Resting Potential**:
   - At rest, a neuron has a **negative charge** inside the cell compared to the outside. This difference in charge is known as the **resting membrane potential** (around -70 mV). The resting potential is maintained by the

sodium-potassium pump, which actively transports sodium ions (Na^+) out of the neuron and potassium ions (K^+) into the neuron.

2. **Depolarization**:
   - When a neuron is stimulated by a signal from another neuron or sensory input, **sodium channels** in the membrane open, allowing sodium ions (Na^+) to rush into the cell. This influx of positively charged sodium ions causes the inside of the neuron to become less negative, or **depolarized**.
   - If the depolarization reaches a certain threshold (approximately -55 mV), an action potential is triggered.
3. **Action Potential**:
   - Once the threshold is reached, the neuron undergoes rapid depolarization, with more sodium channels opening, allowing even more sodium ions to flow into the neuron. The membrane potential briefly becomes **positive** (up to +30 mV).

- This rapid change in charge creates the action potential, an electrical signal that travels down the axon of the neuron.

4. **Repolarization**:
   - After the peak of the action potential is reached, **potassium channels** open, allowing potassium ions (K^+) to flow out of the neuron. This outward movement of positively charged ions helps restore the negative charge inside the cell.
   - This process is known as **repolarization**.

5. **Hyperpolarization and Refractory Period**:
   - The membrane potential temporarily becomes more negative than the resting potential, a state called **hyperpolarization**. This occurs because potassium ions continue to leave the cell after repolarization.
   - During the **refractory period**, the neuron cannot fire another action potential, ensuring the

signal only moves in one direction.

6. **Return to Resting Potential**:
   - The sodium-potassium pump restores the normal distribution of sodium and potassium ions, returning the neuron to its **resting potential**, ready for the next impulse.

Propagation of the Nerve Impulse

The action potential travels along the **axon** of the neuron like a wave. As the action potential moves down the axon, the depolarization in one area causes adjacent areas of the axon membrane to depolarize, creating a chain reaction that carries the signal toward the **axon terminals**.

In **myelinated axons**, the nerve impulse moves much faster due to **saltatory conduction**, where the action potential jumps from one **Node of Ranvier** (gaps in the myelin sheath) to the next, significantly speeding up signal transmission.

Synaptic Transmission

When the nerve impulse reaches the **axon terminals**, it causes the release of neurotransmitters from **synaptic vesicles** into the **synapse** (the gap between neurons). These neurotransmitters cross the synaptic cleft and bind to receptors on the next neuron, stimulating or inhibiting the generation of a new action potential in that cell. This is how nerve impulses are passed from one neuron to the next, allowing the nervous system to coordinate complex functions.

Herbs, Vitamins, Minerals, and Supplements (HVMS) for Nerve Impulse Health

1. **Herbs**:
    - **Ginkgo Biloba**: Known to enhance circulation and improve the delivery of oxygen and nutrients to nerve cells, supporting healthy nerve impulses.
    - **Bacopa Monnieri**: An herb traditionally used in Ayurvedic medicine, bacopa improves cognitive function and supports nerve health, enhancing synaptic transmission.

- **Ashwagandha**: Helps reduce oxidative stress on neurons, preserving nerve impulse function and promoting overall nervous system health.

2. **Vitamins**:
   - **Vitamin B1 (Thiamine)**: Essential for nerve function, thiamine helps maintain the integrity of nerve cell membranes and supports the proper transmission of nerve impulses.
   - **Vitamin B6 (Pyridoxine)**: Plays a critical role in neurotransmitter synthesis, supporting the release of chemicals that transmit signals between neurons.
   - **Vitamin B12 (Cobalamin)**: Important for the production of myelin, the protective sheath around neurons that facilitates the rapid transmission of nerve impulses.

3. **Minerals**:
   - **Magnesium**: Vital for nerve impulse transmission, magnesium helps regulate the movement of ions across cell

membranes, preventing
abnormal nerve firing and
supporting a calm nervous
system.

- **Calcium**: Necessary for the
  release of neurotransmitters at
  synapses, calcium is involved in
  initiating nerve impulses and
  ensuring proper communication
  between neurons.
- **Potassium**: Helps maintain the
  resting membrane potential of
  neurons, ensuring that nerve
  impulses are generated and
  transmitted effectively.

4. **Supplements**:

- **Alpha-Lipoic Acid**: An
  antioxidant that protects nerve
  cells from damage and supports
  the health of the nervous system
  by improving the transmission of
  nerve impulses.
- **Acetyl-L-Carnitine**: Enhances
  energy production in nerve cells
  and supports nerve repair,
  promoting healthy nerve impulse
  conduction.
- **Fish Oil (Omega-3 Fatty
  Acids)**: Contains essential fatty

acids that support the health of myelin and improve nerve cell communication, facilitating efficient nerve impulse transmission.

By understanding the detailed mechanics of nerve impulse transmission and nurturing nerve health through proper nutrition and supplements, you can maintain a healthy nervous system and support the vital functions it controls.

Synapse

A **synapse** is the point of communication between two neurons, or between a neuron and another type of cell (such as a muscle or gland cell). It is a small gap where the electrical signal of a nerve impulse is converted into a chemical signal, allowing neurons to communicate and transmit information across the nervous system. Synapses are critical for processing and transmitting signals, enabling everything from simple reflexes to complex thoughts.

Structure of a Synapse

The synapse consists of three main components:

1. **Presynaptic Neuron**:
    - The neuron that sends the signal. At the end of its **axon terminals**, it contains small vesicles filled with neurotransmitters.
2. **Synaptic Cleft**:
    - The tiny gap (about 20-40 nanometers wide) between the presynaptic and postsynaptic neurons, across which the neurotransmitters must travel.

3. **Postsynaptic Neuron**:
    - The neuron or cell that receives the signal. It has specific **receptor proteins** on its membrane that bind to neurotransmitters.

The Synaptic Transmission Process

Synaptic transmission involves the conversion of the electrical signal (action potential) into a chemical signal and then back into an electrical signal in the receiving neuron. Here's how this process occurs:

1. **Action Potential Arrival**:
    - When an action potential reaches the axon terminal of the presynaptic neuron, it triggers the opening of **voltage-gated calcium channels**. Calcium ions (Ca^{2+}) flow into the presynaptic terminal.
2. **Neurotransmitter Release**:
    - The influx of calcium causes **synaptic vesicles** filled with neurotransmitters (chemical messengers) to fuse with the presynaptic membrane. This fusion releases the

neurotransmitters into the
synaptic cleft.

3. **Neurotransmitter Binding**:
   - The neurotransmitters diffuse across the synaptic cleft and bind to **receptors** on the membrane of the postsynaptic neuron. Each type of neurotransmitter has specific receptors it can bind to.

4. **Postsynaptic Potential**:
   - When neurotransmitters bind to their receptors, they cause changes in the postsynaptic neuron's membrane. This can either **excite** the neuron (by causing depolarization and increasing the likelihood of firing an action potential) or **inhibit** it (by causing hyperpolarization and decreasing the likelihood of firing).
     - **Excitatory neurotransmitters**: Cause the postsynaptic neuron to become more positive (closer to the threshold for firing an action potential).

- **Inhibitory neurotransmitters**: Cause the postsynaptic neuron to become more negative, making it less likely to fire.

5. **Termination of Signal**:
   - Once the signal has been transmitted, the neurotransmitters are quickly removed from the synaptic cleft. This can happen through:
     - **Reuptake**: Neurotransmitters are taken back up into the presynaptic neuron.
     - **Enzymatic Degradation**: Enzymes break down the neurotransmitters in the synaptic cleft.
     - **Diffusion**: Neurotransmitters drift away from the synapse.

6. **Signal Propagation**:
   - If the signal is excitatory and the postsynaptic neuron reaches the threshold, it will generate a new

action potential, continuing the transmission of the signal.

Types of Synapses

- **Electrical Synapse**: In an electrical synapse, the electrical signal passes directly from one neuron to the next through **gap junctions**, without the need for neurotransmitters. These synapses are rare in humans but are found in specific brain regions and allow for rapid communication.
- **Chemical Synapse**: The most common type, where neurotransmitters are used to relay signals. Chemical synapses allow for more complex processing and modulation of signals compared to electrical synapses.

Key Neurotransmitters

- **Acetylcholine (ACh)**: Involved in muscle activation, learning, and memory.
- **Dopamine**: Regulates mood, motivation, and reward.
- **Serotonin**: Plays a role in mood regulation, sleep, and appetite.

- **Gamma-Aminobutyric Acid (GABA)**: The primary inhibitory neurotransmitter in the brain, reducing neuronal excitability.
- **Glutamate**: The primary excitatory neurotransmitter, critical for learning and memory.

Herbs, Vitamins, Minerals, and Supplements (HVMS) for Synapse Health

1. **Herbs**:
   - **Ginkgo Biloba**: Enhances synaptic plasticity and supports the formation of new synapses, boosting memory and cognitive function.
   - **Lion's Mane Mushroom**: Promotes nerve growth factor (NGF), which supports the repair and development of synapses, aiding learning and memory.
   - **Gotu Kola**: Known for its neuroprotective effects, it can enhance synaptic strength and aid in cognitive performance.
2. **Vitamins**:

- **Vitamin B6**: Plays a key role in neurotransmitter synthesis, helping maintain synaptic function.
  - **Vitamin D**: Supports synaptic plasticity and can influence cognitive processes.
  - **Vitamin B12**: Critical for the maintenance of the myelin sheath and overall nerve health, facilitating effective synaptic transmission.
3. **Minerals**:
   - **Magnesium**: Essential for synaptic transmission, particularly in preventing the overexcitation of neurons and maintaining a balanced signal.
   - **Zinc**: Involved in neurotransmitter release and synaptic plasticity, zinc plays a role in memory formation.
   - **Calcium**: Key to triggering neurotransmitter release from presynaptic terminals.
4. **Supplements**:
   - **Omega-3 Fatty Acids (DHA/EPA)**: Support synaptic function and structure,

promoting neurogenesis and protecting against cognitive decline.

- **N-Acetyl Cysteine (NAC)**: An antioxidant that aids in reducing oxidative stress on synapses, preserving their function.
- **Phosphatidylserine**: Important for maintaining the integrity of synaptic membranes, enhancing memory, and improving cognitive function.

By understanding the science of synaptic function and nourishing these essential structures with targeted nutrients, you can optimize your brain's communication pathways and support overall mental health.

Myelin

Myelin is a fatty, white substance that forms a sheath around the axons of neurons, acting as an insulating layer. This insulation is essential for the efficient transmission of electrical signals (action potentials) along the nerve fibers. Myelin is produced by two types of glial cells: **Schwann cells** in the **peripheral nervous system (PNS)** and **oligodendrocytes** in the **central nervous system (CNS)**.

Structure and Function of Myelin

1. **Insulation and Signal Transmission**:
   - Myelin wraps around the axons in a spiral fashion, creating multiple layers of membrane. This insulation prevents the loss of electrical current and allows the nerve impulse to travel much faster compared to unmyelinated axons.
   - The gaps between myelinated segments, known as **Nodes of Ranvier**, allow the action potential to "jump" from node to node in a process called **saltatory conduction**, greatly

increasing the speed of neural communication.

2. **Protection**:
   - Myelin also protects the axons from external damage and helps maintain the overall health of the neurons.

3. **Energy Efficiency**:
   - By allowing the signal to travel quickly, myelin reduces the amount of energy neurons need to expend to transmit impulses, conserving cellular resources.

The Importance of Myelination

Myelination is critical for proper nervous system function. The process begins in fetal development and continues into adulthood, peaking during childhood and adolescence as the nervous system matures. Proper myelination is essential for motor skills, sensory processing, cognitive functions, and coordination.

When myelin is damaged or degraded, as in diseases like **multiple sclerosis (MS)**, the efficiency of nerve signal transmission is severely reduced, leading to a range of neurological symptoms, such as muscle weakness, fatigue, coordination problems, and impaired cognitive function.

Demyelination

Demyelination is the process by which the myelin sheath is damaged or lost. This can occur due to autoimmune diseases (such as multiple sclerosis), infections, genetic mutations, or toxins. Demyelination can slow down or block nerve impulses, leading to various neurological disorders and symptoms like numbness, paralysis, vision problems, and impaired motor control.

Key Roles of Myelin:

- **Fast Signal Transmission**: Enables rapid communication between neurons and across long distances in the body.
- **Neuroprotection**: Shields axons from physical damage and neurotoxins.
- **Efficient Energy Use**: Reduces the energy demands on neurons by speeding up signal propagation.

Herbs, Vitamins, Minerals, and Supplements (HVMS) for Myelin Health

1. **Herbs**:
    - **Gotu Kola**: Known to enhance myelination and support nerve regeneration, aiding in the repair and protection of the myelin sheath.
    - **Lion's Mane Mushroom**: Stimulates the production of nerve growth factor (NGF), which supports the maintenance and repair of myelin.
    - **Ashwagandha**: Has neuroprotective properties and may help promote myelin repair and nerve health.
2. **Vitamins**:
    - **Vitamin B12**: Crucial for maintaining the health of the myelin sheath. A deficiency in B12 can lead to demyelination and nervous system disorders.
    - **Vitamin D**: Supports immune function and may help prevent autoimmune attacks on the myelin sheath.
    - **Folate (Vitamin B9)**: Involved in the synthesis of neurotransmitters and maintenance of the nervous

system, helping to protect the myelin sheath.

3. **Minerals**:
    - **Magnesium**: Supports overall nerve function and has a calming effect on the nervous system, which may protect against nerve damage.
    - **Zinc**: Plays a role in myelin repair and regeneration, supporting the production of proteins essential for nerve health.
    - **Iron**: Required for proper nerve function and myelination, particularly during development.
4. **Supplements**:
    - **Omega-3 Fatty Acids (DHA/EPA)**: Essential for the structure of the myelin sheath. These fatty acids are integral to nerve cell membranes and help maintain and repair myelin.
    - **Phosphatidylserine**: A phospholipid that supports the structure of nerve cells and aids in maintaining the integrity of myelin.

- **Acetyl-L-Carnitine**: Known for its neuroprotective effects, it may help promote the repair of damaged myelin and improve cognitive function.

By understanding the role of myelin in nerve function and utilizing the right combination of nutrients, herbs, and supplements, you can support the maintenance and repair of this essential component of the nervous system, promoting overall neurological health and resilience.

Dopamine

Dopamine is a crucial neurotransmitter in the brain that plays a significant role in various functions, including movement, motivation, reward, and pleasure. It is produced in several areas of the brain, most notably the **substantia nigra** and the **ventral tegmental area**. Dopamine influences behavior, mood, cognition, attention, and even learning. Imbalances in dopamine levels are associated with various conditions, such as **Parkinson's disease**, **schizophrenia**, and **addiction**.

Functions of Dopamine

1. **Reward and Pleasure:**
   - Dopamine is best known for its role in the brain's reward system. When you experience something pleasurable, such as eating, achieving a goal, or social interaction, dopamine is released, creating feelings of satisfaction and reinforcing the behavior.
2. **Motivation:**
   - It helps drive behaviors by providing the motivation to pursue goals and rewards. High levels of dopamine increase

motivation and focus, while low levels can result in apathy and lack of interest in daily activities.

3. **Motor Control**:
   - Dopamine is involved in coordinating movement. In the **basal ganglia**, dopamine regulates motor control, and its deficiency leads to motor disorders like Parkinson's disease, characterized by tremors, stiffness, and slow movements.
4. **Cognitive Function**:
   - Dopamine affects various cognitive functions, including attention, working memory, and learning. It helps regulate the brain circuits involved in decision-making and problem-solving.
5. **Emotional Regulation**:
   - Dopamine is involved in mood regulation. Imbalances in dopamine levels can contribute to mood disorders like depression, anxiety, or mania.

Dopaminergic Pathways

There are several key pathways in the brain where dopamine plays a vital role:

1. **Mesolimbic Pathway**:
    - Often referred to as the "reward pathway," it is associated with pleasure, reinforcement learning, and addiction. Dopamine release in this pathway reinforces pleasurable experiences.
2. **Nigrostriatal Pathway**:
    - Involved in movement and motor control, degeneration of dopamine neurons in this pathway is a hallmark of Parkinson's disease.
3. **Mesocortical Pathway**:
    - Linked to cognitive functions, attention, and emotional responses. This pathway is associated with schizophrenia and other cognitive and emotional disorders.
4. **Tuberoinfundibular Pathway**:
    - Inhibits the release of **prolactin**, a hormone involved in lactation. Dopamine from this pathway regulates endocrine function.

Dopamine Deficiency and Excess

- **Deficiency**: Low levels of dopamine can result in lack of motivation, fatigue, depression, and motor control problems (e.g., Parkinson's). Cognitive impairments such as difficulty concentrating or making decisions are also common.
- **Excess**: Excessive dopamine can lead to conditions such as schizophrenia, which involves hallucinations, delusions, and hyperactivity. It is also linked to impulsive behaviors and addiction, as overstimulation of the reward system drives compulsive behavior.

Herbs, Vitamins, Minerals, and Supplements (HVMS) to Support Dopamine Production

1. **Herbs**:
    - **Mucuna Pruriens**: Contains **L-DOPA**, a direct precursor to dopamine, helping boost dopamine levels naturally. Often used in herbal treatments for Parkinson's.
    - **Ginkgo Biloba**: Enhances blood flow to the brain, supporting overall cognitive function and

potentially increasing dopamine availability.

- **Rhodiola Rosea**: An adaptogen that helps balance stress and improve mood by modulating dopamine levels.

2. **Vitamins**:

- **Vitamin B6 (Pyridoxine)**: Involved in the synthesis of dopamine from L-DOPA, making it essential for dopamine production.
- **Vitamin C**: Plays a role in converting dopamine into norepinephrine, maintaining dopamine balance in the brain.
- **Folate (Vitamin B9)**: Supports the creation of neurotransmitters, including dopamine, by assisting in the methylation process.

3. **Minerals**:

- **Magnesium**: Supports the proper functioning of the brain's dopamine receptors, contributing to balanced mood and mental well-being.
- **Zinc**: Essential for dopamine signaling and regulation, a

deficiency in zinc can lead to issues with mood and cognition.
  - **Iron**: Required for the conversion of tyrosine into dopamine, making it a critical component in dopamine production.

4. **Supplements**:
  - **L-Tyrosine**: An amino acid that is a direct precursor to dopamine, it can help boost dopamine levels and improve cognitive performance under stress.
  - **Acetyl-L-Carnitine (ALCAR)**: Promotes mental clarity and energy by supporting dopamine synthesis and its receptors.
  - **Phosphatidylserine**: A phospholipid that enhances brain function, including dopamine release, and improves memory and cognition.

Dopamine is integral to mental health, motor control, and emotional well-being. By incorporating the right herbs, vitamins, minerals, and supplements, you can naturally support dopamine production and maintain balanced neurological health, motivation, and emotional stability.

Serotonin

Serotonin is a critical neurotransmitter that plays a significant role in regulating mood, sleep, digestion, and overall well-being. It is synthesized in the brain and the intestines, with around 90% of serotonin found in the gastrointestinal tract, where it regulates bowel movements, and the remaining 10% in the brain, where it influences mood and behavior.

Functions of Serotonin

1. **Mood Regulation**:
    - Serotonin is often referred to as the "feel-good" neurotransmitter because of its strong influence on mood. It helps stabilize emotions, contributing to feelings of happiness and well-being. Low serotonin levels are associated with depression, anxiety, and mood disorders.
2. **Sleep**:
    - Serotonin is a precursor to **melatonin**, the hormone that regulates sleep-wake cycles. It helps in falling asleep and maintaining a restful sleep pattern.

3. **Digestion**:
    - In the gut, serotonin regulates intestinal movements and can influence appetite, nausea, and bowel function. It helps modulate digestion by ensuring proper contraction of the intestines.
4. **Cognitive Function**:
    - Serotonin impacts learning, memory, and cognitive processing. Balanced serotonin levels promote focus and clarity, while deficiencies can affect attention and cognitive function.
5. **Sexual Function**:
    - It has a regulatory effect on libido and sexual desire. Imbalances in serotonin levels can affect sexual function, often reducing libido when levels are high and increasing it when they are low.
6. **Blood Clotting**:
    - Serotonin is released by platelets during the clotting process. It causes blood vessels to narrow, aiding in clot formation.
7. **Bone Health**:
    - Research suggests that serotonin plays a role in bone density

regulation, with high levels of circulating serotonin potentially contributing to lower bone mass.

Serotonin Pathways

- **Central Nervous System (CNS):** In the brain, serotonin regulates mood, anxiety, and sleep. It acts on various parts of the brain, including the **hippocampus** (memory), **amygdala** (emotions), and **prefrontal cortex** (cognitive function).
- **Peripheral Nervous System (PNS):** In the gut, serotonin controls digestion and is involved in bowel movements and peristalsis. It also helps regulate nausea and appetite.

Serotonin Deficiency and Excess

- **Deficiency:** Low serotonin levels are linked to several disorders, including **depression, anxiety, insomnia**, and **irritable bowel syndrome** (IBS). Symptoms can include mood swings, difficulty sleeping, fatigue, and changes in appetite.
- **Excess:** Excess serotonin can lead to **serotonin syndrome**, a potentially life-threatening condition that occurs

when too much serotonin builds up in the brain. It is characterized by symptoms such as confusion, agitation, rapid heart rate, and muscle rigidity. This can be caused by certain medications, especially antidepressants.

Herbs, Vitamins, Minerals, and Supplements (HVMS) to Support Serotonin Production

1. **Herbs**:
   - **St. John's Wort**: Often used for mild to moderate depression, it is believed to increase serotonin levels by inhibiting serotonin reuptake.
   - **Saffron**: Known for its mood-enhancing properties, saffron may boost serotonin levels and improve symptoms of depression and anxiety.
   - **Rhodiola Rosea**: An adaptogen that helps reduce stress and anxiety, it is thought to support serotonin balance and improve mood stability.

- o **Ginseng**: Helps reduce stress and fatigue, promoting overall mental clarity and possibly boosting serotonin levels.

2. **Vitamins**:
    - o **Vitamin B6**: Essential for the conversion of **tryptophan** into serotonin, B6 plays a crucial role in serotonin production.
    - o **Vitamin D**: Low levels of vitamin D are linked to decreased serotonin production, and supplementation may help enhance mood and energy.
    - o **Folate (Vitamin B9)**: Supports the production of serotonin by assisting in the synthesis of neurotransmitters, especially in individuals with folate deficiencies.
    - o **Vitamin C**: Though more commonly associated with immune support, vitamin C also plays a role in neurotransmitter function, including serotonin.

3. **Minerals**:
    - o **Magnesium**: Magnesium helps activate serotonin receptors in the brain. Deficiency in

magnesium is linked to increased symptoms of depression and anxiety.

- **Zinc**: Zinc is essential for brain function and neurotransmitter regulation, and low levels are associated with depressive symptoms. It supports serotonin signaling.
- **Calcium**: Calcium is needed for serotonin metabolism and helps maintain the stability of mood and overall brain function.

4. **Supplements**:
   - **5-HTP (5-Hydroxytryptophan)**: A direct precursor to serotonin, 5-HTP is often used to boost serotonin levels and improve mood, sleep, and reduce symptoms of depression.
   - **L-Tryptophan**: An essential amino acid, tryptophan is converted into serotonin in the brain. Supplementation can increase serotonin levels, helping to stabilize mood and promote relaxation.

- **Omega-3 Fatty Acids**: Found in fish oil, omega-3 fatty acids help enhance serotonin transmission in the brain, improving overall mental health.
- **Probiotics**: Probiotics that support gut health, such as **Lactobacillus** and **Bifidobacterium**, may also promote serotonin production, as the majority of serotonin is produced in the gut.

Serotonin is vital for maintaining mental, emotional, and physical health. By incorporating the right herbs, vitamins, minerals, and supplements, you can naturally support serotonin production, balance mood, enhance sleep, and improve overall well-being.

Acetylcholine

Acetylcholine (ACh) is a vital neurotransmitter in both the central and peripheral nervous systems, playing crucial roles in numerous physiological processes. Discovered in the early 20th century, it is the first neurotransmitter identified and remains one of the most studied due to its significance in various bodily functions.

Functions of Acetylcholine

1. **Neuromuscular Transmission:**
   - ACh is essential for muscle contraction. It is released from motor neurons at the neuromuscular junction, binding to receptors on muscle fibers and triggering contractions. This action is vital for all voluntary muscle movements, from walking to breathing.
2. **Central Nervous System Activity:**
   - In the brain, acetylcholine modulates various cognitive functions, including attention, learning, memory, and arousal. It plays a critical role in enhancing sensory perception and is

involved in the encoding of memories, especially in the hippocampus.

3. **Autonomic Nervous System**:
   - ACh functions in the autonomic nervous system (ANS), which regulates involuntary bodily functions. It is a key neurotransmitter in the parasympathetic nervous system, promoting "rest and digest" activities. It slows the heart rate, increases digestive secretions, and stimulates peristalsis in the intestines.

4. **Sleep Regulation**:
   - Acetylcholine is involved in the regulation of sleep, particularly the REM (rapid eye movement) phase, where dreaming occurs. Its levels fluctuate during the sleep cycle, contributing to the modulation of sleep states.

5. **Pain Perception**:
   - It plays a role in pain signaling pathways and can affect how pain is perceived by the brain, influencing both the sensory and emotional components of pain.

6. **Cognitive Function**:
    - ACh is crucial for attention and focus. Enhanced acetylcholine activity can improve cognitive performance, while reduced levels are associated with cognitive decline and disorders such as Alzheimer's disease.

Acetylcholine Receptors

Acetylcholine acts on two primary types of receptors:

1. **Nicotinic Receptors**:
    - These receptors are ionotropic and mediate fast synaptic transmission. They are found at the neuromuscular junction and in the central nervous system, playing a significant role in muscle contraction and cognitive functions.
2. **Muscarinic Receptors**:
    - These are metabotropic receptors that mediate slower, modulatory effects. They are primarily found in the brain and various peripheral tissues, including the heart and digestive system,

contributing to the parasympathetic nervous system's functions.

Acetylcholine Synthesis and Breakdown

- **Synthesis**: Acetylcholine is synthesized from acetyl-CoA and choline, a nutrient that can be obtained from dietary sources like eggs, fish, and nuts.
- **Release and Action**: Upon the arrival of an action potential, ACh is released into the synaptic cleft and binds to its receptors on the postsynaptic membrane, facilitating neurotransmission.
- **Degradation**: After exerting its effect, acetylcholine is rapidly broken down by the enzyme **acetylcholinesterase** into acetate and choline, terminating its action and allowing the neuron to reset for the next signal.

Acetylcholine Deficiency and Excess

- **Deficiency**: Low levels of acetylcholine are associated with cognitive decline, memory loss, and conditions like Alzheimer's disease. Symptoms can include confusion, difficulty concentrating, and impaired muscle function.

- **Excess**: High levels of acetylcholine can lead to overstimulation of the nervous system, causing symptoms such as muscle cramps, spasms, or even paralysis. It may also result in excessive salivation, sweating, and gastrointestinal distress.

Herbs, Vitamins, Minerals, and Supplements (HVMS) to Support Acetylcholine Production

1. **Herbs**:
    - **Ginkgo Biloba**: Known for improving cognitive function and memory, it may enhance blood flow to the brain, supporting acetylcholine levels and receptor sensitivity.
    - **Bacopa Monnieri**: An adaptogen used in traditional medicine, it has been shown to improve memory and cognitive function by potentially increasing acetylcholine levels.

- **Huperzine A**: Derived from the Chinese club moss, it inhibits acetylcholinesterase, increasing acetylcholine levels and improving memory and learning.
- **Rhodiola Rosea**: An adaptogen that may support cognitive function and stress management, possibly enhancing acetylcholine release.

2. **Vitamins**:

- **Vitamin B5 (Pantothenic Acid)**: Essential for the synthesis of acetylcholine, a deficiency may impair its production.
- **Vitamin B1 (Thiamine)**: Supports neurotransmitter synthesis and may help improve cognitive function and mental clarity.
- **Vitamin B6 (Pyridoxine)**: Plays a crucial role in the synthesis of neurotransmitters, including acetylcholine.
- **Vitamin B12 (Cobalamin)**: Supports nerve health and function, contributing to proper neurotransmission.

3. **Minerals**:

- **Choline**: A precursor to acetylcholine, sufficient intake is necessary for optimal neurotransmitter synthesis. Sources include eggs, liver, and soybeans.
  - **Magnesium**: Supports overall nervous system function and may help regulate acetylcholine release, impacting muscle function and cognitive health.

4. **Supplements**:
   - **Alpha-GPC (L-alpha glycerylphosphorylcholine)**: A choline compound that crosses the blood-brain barrier, promoting acetylcholine synthesis and enhancing cognitive performance.
   - **CDP-Choline (Citicoline)**: A choline source that supports cognitive function and may improve memory by enhancing acetylcholine levels.
   - **Acetyl-L-Carnitine**: An amino acid that may support mitochondrial function and enhance acetylcholine levels,

improving cognitive performance and mood.

- **Phosphatidylserine**: A phospholipid that supports cell membrane integrity and may enhance acetylcholine release, promoting cognitive function.

Acetylcholine is a key player in numerous physiological functions, from muscle contraction to cognitive processes. By supporting its synthesis and action through appropriate herbs, vitamins, minerals, and supplements, you can enhance your overall brain health and physical performance.

GABA

Gamma-aminobutyric acid (GABA) is a crucial neurotransmitter in the central nervous system, known primarily for its role as the primary inhibitory neurotransmitter in the brain. Discovered in the 1950s, GABA has garnered significant attention for its calming effects on neural activity and its potential therapeutic applications in various neurological and psychological conditions.

Functions of GABA

1. **Inhibition of Neuronal Activity:**
   - GABA's primary function is to inhibit or reduce neuronal excitability throughout the nervous system. It binds to GABA receptors on the postsynaptic neurons, causing an influx of chloride ions (Cl^-) or an efflux of potassium ions (K^+), resulting in hyperpolarization of the neuron and making it less likely to fire. This mechanism is essential for maintaining the balance between excitation and inhibition in the brain.
2. **Regulation of Anxiety and Stress:**

- By reducing neuronal excitability, GABA plays a key role in modulating anxiety and stress responses. It helps create a sense of calm and relaxation, counteracting the effects of excitatory neurotransmitters like glutamate.

3. **Sleep Regulation**:
   - GABA is crucial for promoting sleep and regulating the sleep-wake cycle. It helps to initiate and maintain sleep by inhibiting neural activity associated with wakefulness, leading to deeper and more restful sleep.

4. **Muscle Relaxation**:
   - GABA also plays a role in muscle tone regulation. It can inhibit motor neuron activity, leading to muscle relaxation. This is particularly important in preventing excessive muscle contractions and spasms.

5. **Neuroprotection**:
   - GABA may exert neuroprotective effects by preventing excitotoxicity, a condition where

excessive neuronal activation leads to cell death. By inhibiting overactivity, GABA helps protect neurons from damage, particularly in conditions like stroke and neurodegenerative diseases.

6. **Role in Cognitive Function**:
    o   While primarily inhibitory, GABA is also involved in cognitive processes, including attention, memory, and learning. Its balance with excitatory neurotransmitters is crucial for optimal cognitive function.

GABA Receptors

GABA acts on two primary types of receptors:

1. **GABAA_AA Receptors**:
    o   These are ionotropic receptors that mediate fast synaptic inhibition. When GABA binds to GABAA_AA receptors, it opens chloride channels, resulting in rapid hyperpolarization of the neuron. These receptors are the targets of several anxiolytic (anxiety-reducing) medications,

including benzodiazepines, which enhance GABA's inhibitory effects.

2. **GABAB_BB Receptors**:
   - These are metabotropic receptors that mediate slower, prolonged inhibitory effects through G-protein coupled signaling. Activation of GABAB_BB receptors can inhibit neurotransmitter release and modulate neuronal excitability over longer periods.

GABA Synthesis and Breakdown

- **Synthesis**: GABA is synthesized from glutamate, an excitatory neurotransmitter, through the action of the enzyme **glutamic acid decarboxylase (GAD)**, which requires vitamin B6 (pyridoxine) as a cofactor. This process highlights the interplay between excitatory and inhibitory neurotransmission in the brain.
- **Release and Action**: Upon the arrival of an action potential, GABA is released into the synaptic cleft, where it binds to its receptors on the postsynaptic membrane, inhibiting neuronal firing.

- **Reuptake and Breakdown**: GABA's action is terminated by reuptake into the presynaptic neuron or surrounding glial cells, primarily via the GABA transporter. Once inside the cell, GABA can be converted back to glutamate or metabolized by enzymes like GABA transaminase.

GABA Deficiency and Excess

- **Deficiency**: Low levels of GABA have been linked to various conditions, including anxiety disorders, depression, insomnia, epilepsy, and muscle spasms. Symptoms may include increased anxiety, restlessness, insomnia, and heightened sensitivity to stress.
- **Excess**: While GABA is primarily inhibitory, excessive GABA activity can lead to over-sedation, cognitive impairment, and impaired motor function. This can occur with the use of GABAergic medications or substances that enhance GABA activity.

Herbs, Vitamins, Minerals, and Supplements (HVMS) to Support GABA Production

1. **Herbs**:
   - **Valerian Root**: Known for its sedative properties, valerian may enhance GABA activity, promoting relaxation and improving sleep quality.
   - **Passionflower**: This herb is often used for its calming effects and may increase GABA levels, helping to reduce anxiety and improve sleep.
   - **L-theanine**: An amino acid found in tea leaves, it can promote relaxation and increase GABA levels, enhancing mood and reducing stress.
   - **Kava**: Traditionally used for its anxiolytic effects, kava may enhance GABAergic activity, promoting relaxation without sedation.
2. **Vitamins**:
   - **Vitamin B6 (Pyridoxine)**: Crucial for the synthesis of GABA from glutamate, adequate levels

of B6 are necessary for optimal GABA production.

- **Vitamin B12 (Cobalamin):** Supports overall nervous system function and may contribute to maintaining healthy GABA levels.

3. **Minerals:**

- **Magnesium:** This mineral plays a role in the regulation of GABA receptors, and deficiency may lead to increased excitability and anxiety.
- **Zinc:** Involved in neurotransmitter synthesis and regulation, zinc may support healthy GABA levels and receptor function.

4. **Supplements:**

- **GABA Supplements:** While some debate exists regarding the effectiveness of supplemental GABA crossing the blood-brain barrier, many individuals report calming effects from these products.
- **L-Theanine:** As mentioned, this amino acid can promote relaxation and increase GABA

levels, making it a popular supplement for stress relief.

- **Ashwagandha**: An adaptogenic herb that may help regulate GABA levels and support stress management and anxiety reduction.
- **5-HTP (5-Hydroxytryptophan)**: While primarily a serotonin precursor, 5-HTP may indirectly support GABA levels by promoting overall neurotransmitter balance.

GABA is a key neurotransmitter that plays a vital role in promoting calm, relaxation, and overall mental well-being. By supporting GABA production and activity through appropriate herbs, vitamins, minerals, and supplements, individuals can enhance their emotional resilience and improve their quality of life.

Reflex Arc

The **reflex arc** is a fundamental neural pathway that mediates reflex actions, allowing for rapid responses to stimuli without the need for conscious thought. This mechanism is crucial for protecting the body from harm and maintaining homeostasis. It comprises several key components that work together to facilitate swift reflex actions, often referred to as "reflexes."

Components of the Reflex Arc

1. **Receptor:**
    - The reflex arc begins with a **receptor**, which is a specialized nerve ending that detects a specific stimulus. This can be anything from heat, pressure, pain, or stretch. When the receptor is stimulated, it converts the sensory input into an electrical signal (nerve impulse).
2. **Sensory Neuron:**
    - The electrical signal travels along a **sensory neuron**, which transmits the impulse from the receptor to the spinal cord or brainstem. This neuron is

responsible for conveying information about the stimulus to the central nervous system (CNS).

3. **Integration Center**:
   - Within the spinal cord or brain, the impulse reaches an **integration center** (often a simple synapse in the spinal cord for reflexes). Here, the sensory neuron communicates with one or more interneurons or directly with motor neurons, depending on the complexity of the reflex. The integration center processes the information and generates an appropriate response.

4. **Motor Neuron**:
   - Once the integration center has processed the information, a **motor neuron** transmits the response signal from the CNS to the effector. This neuron carries the impulse away from the spinal cord to the target organ or muscle.

5. **Effector**:
   - The pathway concludes at the **effector**, which can be a muscle

or a gland. Upon receiving the signal from the motor neuron, the effector performs the necessary action, such as contracting a muscle to withdraw a hand from a hot surface or secreting a substance from a gland.

Types of Reflex Arcs

Reflex arcs can be categorized based on their complexity and the number of synapses involved:

1. **Monosynaptic Reflex Arc**:
   - This type of reflex arc involves a single synapse between a sensory neuron and a motor neuron. The **patellar reflex** (knee-jerk reaction) is a classic example, where tapping the patellar tendon stimulates the quadriceps muscle to contract.
2. **Polysynaptic Reflex Arc**:
   - This reflex arc includes one or more interneurons between the sensory and motor neurons, allowing for more complex responses. An example is the **withdrawal reflex**, where

multiple muscles are activated to withdraw a limb from a painful stimulus, requiring coordination among several muscle groups.

Function and Importance of the Reflex Arc

The reflex arc is essential for several reasons:

- **Rapid Response**: Reflexes occur quickly, often before the brain has a chance to process the stimulus consciously. This rapid response is vital for survival, allowing the body to react swiftly to harmful stimuli, such as touching a hot surface.
- **Protection**: Reflex arcs play a crucial role in protective mechanisms, safeguarding the body from injury. For example, the withdrawal reflex prevents further tissue damage by quickly moving the body away from harmful stimuli.
- **Homeostasis**: Reflex arcs contribute to maintaining homeostasis by regulating bodily functions, such as heart rate, blood pressure, and digestion. For instance, baroreceptors detect changes in blood pressure and trigger reflex responses to adjust heart rate and vascular tone.

Herbs, Vitamins, Minerals, and Supplements (HVMS) for Supporting the Reflex Arc

Herbs

1. **Ginkgo Biloba**: Known for improving blood circulation and enhancing cognitive function, which can support neural communication.
2. **Ashwagandha**: An adaptogen that helps reduce stress and anxiety, potentially improving overall nervous system function.
3. **Rhodiola Rosea**: Helps combat fatigue and enhances physical and mental performance, promoting overall nerve health.
4. **Skullcap**: A calming herb that may help reduce anxiety and improve nervous system function.

Vitamins

1. **Vitamin B1 (Thiamine)**: Essential for nerve function and energy metabolism in nerve cells.

2. **Vitamin B6 (Pyridoxine)**: Plays a crucial role in neurotransmitter synthesis and nerve function.
3. **Vitamin B12 (Cobalamin)**: Vital for maintaining healthy nerve cells and producing DNA and RNA.
4. **Vitamin D**: Supports nerve health and may protect against neurodegeneration.

Minerals

1. **Magnesium**: Critical for nerve transmission and muscle contraction, magnesium supports overall neuromuscular function.
2. **Calcium**: Necessary for neurotransmitter release and muscle contraction; plays a role in excitatory and inhibitory signaling in nerves.
3. **Potassium**: Helps maintain electrical gradients across nerve cells, which is essential for proper nerve impulse conduction.
4. **Zinc**: Important for synaptic function and neurotransmission, zinc supports overall nervous system health.

Supplements

1. **Omega-3 Fatty Acids**: Essential for maintaining the structure of cell membranes and promoting optimal nerve function and communication.
2. **Alpha-Lipoic Acid**: An antioxidant that helps protect nerve tissues from damage and supports overall nerve health.
3. **Acetyl-L-Carnitine**: May enhance cognitive function and support nerve regeneration.
4. **N-Acetyl Cysteine (NAC)**: A powerful antioxidant that helps protect against oxidative stress in the nervous system.

Summary of the Nervous System

The nervous system is a complex network that plays a crucial role in coordinating and regulating body functions. It is divided into two main parts: the Central Nervous System (CNS) and the Peripheral Nervous System (PNS).

Central Nervous System (CNS)

The CNS consists of the brain and spinal cord. It is the primary control center for processing information, controlling voluntary and involuntary actions, and facilitating communication throughout the body. The brain is further divided into three main regions: the cerebrum, cerebellum, and brainstem, each responsible for various functions such as cognition, coordination, and basic life processes. The spinal cord serves as a pathway for signals between the brain and the rest of the body.

Peripheral Nervous System (PNS)

The PNS connects the CNS to the limbs and organs. It is subdivided into the somatic nervous system, which governs voluntary movements, and the autonomic nervous system (ANS), which regulates involuntary functions. The ANS is further divided into the sympathetic nervous system (responsible for the "fight or flight" response) and the parasympathetic nervous system (which promotes "rest and digest" activities).

Neurons and Nerve Impulses

Neurons are the fundamental units of the nervous system, responsible for transmitting signals throughout the body. Each neuron consists of a cell body (soma), dendrites (which receive signals), and an axon (which transmits signals). Nerve impulses are electrical signals that travel along neurons, and they are facilitated by myelin, a fatty substance that insulates axons and speeds up signal transmission.

Neurotransmitters

Chemical messengers called neurotransmitters, such as dopamine, serotonin, acetylcholine, and GABA, play key roles in communication between neurons. They are released at synapses (the junctions between neurons) and influence various physiological processes, including mood, cognition, and muscle contraction.

Reflex Arc

The reflex arc is a fundamental neural pathway that enables quick responses to stimuli without the need for conscious thought. It involves sensory receptors, sensory neurons, interneurons in the spinal cord, motor neurons, and effectors (muscles or glands). This mechanism allows for rapid reactions, such as pulling away from a hot surface.

In conclusion, the nervous system is vital for maintaining homeostasis and enabling interactions with the environment. Understanding its structure and function can help in identifying ways to support and enhance nervous system health through lifestyle choices and appropriate supplementation.

Meet the Author

Hey everyone, just wanted to invite everyone to join me on my social pages. Links below!

Facebook Page....Luna Parnell's Written Works

Patreon page.... patreon.com/Lunastreasures